THURROCK TECHNICAL COLLEGE

SICKLE CELL DISEASE

Ian Franklin is Consultant Haematologist at the Queen Elizabeth Hospital, Birmingham. He specializes in the care of sickle cell patients and works in conjunction with the Birmingham Sickle Cell Service which provides a community service for patients.

*Some other Faber health titles*

THE FERTILITY AND CONTRACEPTION BOOK
*Julia Mosse and Josephine Heaton*

ALZHEIMER'S DISEASE: THE LONG BEREAVEMENT
*Elizabeth Forsythe*

MULTIPLE SCLEROSIS: EXPLORING SICKNESS AND HEALTH
*Elizabeth Forsythe*

SLEEP AND DREAMING *Jacob Empson*

DRUG USE AND ABUSE *James Willis*

FOOD FACTS AND FIGURES *Jill Davies and John Dickerson*

UNDERSTANDING YOUR CHILD *Richard Woolfson*

EVERYWOMAN: A GYNAECOLOGICAL GUIDE FOR LIFE
Fifth Edition *Derek Llewellyn-Jones*

FABER POCKET MEDICAL DICTIONARY *Elizabeth Forsythe*

CERVICAL CANCER *Judith Harvey, Sue Mack and Julian Woolfson*

SAFER SEX *Peter Gordon and Louise Mitchell*

ANOREXIA NERVOSA: THE BROKEN CIRCLE *Ann Erichsen*

AGORAPHOBIA *Ruth Hurst Voce*

YOUR CHILD'S HEALTH *Ivan Blumenthal*

# SICKLE CELL DISEASE

## A Guide for Health Workers, Patients and Carers

IAN FRANKLIN
PhD, MRCP, MRCPath

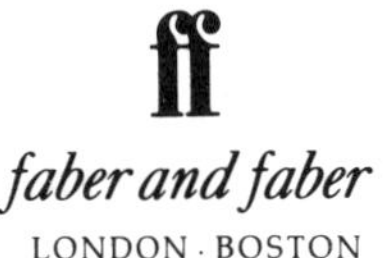

*faber and faber*
LONDON · BOSTON

First published in 1990
by Faber and Faber Limited
3 Queen Square London WC1N 3AU
Photoset by Parker Typesetting Service Leicester
Printed in Great Britain by
Richard Clay Ltd Bungay Suffolk

All rights reserved

© Ian Franklin, 1990

Ian Franklin is hereby identified as author
of this work in accordance with Section 77
of the Copyright, Design and Patents Act 1988.

*This book is sold subject to the condition that it shall not, by way of trade or otherwise, be lent, resold, hired out or otherwise circulated without the publisher's prior consent in any form of binding or cover other than that in which it is published and without a similar condition including this condition being imposed on the subsequent purchaser*

A CIP record for this book is available from the British Library.

ISBN 0 571 14232 X

# Contents

# Preface

I hope that this small book will prove useful to anyone who has an interest in sickle cell disease. In particular I have in mind the nursing, social work and counselling staff who are so important to the effective management of this increasing problem. Some of the chapters have had to be made rather technical and these I hope will appeal and be useful to junior doctors who are perhaps meeting patients with sickle cell disease for the first time. Finally I hope it will also be read by sufferers of sickle cell disease themselves and those who care for them when they are unwell.

I am very grateful to colleagues who have read the manuscript for me, in particular John Stuart, Cage Johnson and David Rogers. I am also extremely grateful to my secretary, Margaret Day, who has consistently managed to produce the typewritten document on schedule.

# Glossary

**Amnesia**
Loss of memory. Absence of recall.

**Amniocentesis**
Removal of fluids surrounding a baby in the womb: enables diagnosis to be made before birth.

**Anaemia**
Low level of haemoglobin in the blood associated with tiredness and lethargy.

**Anaesthetic**
Substance or procedure that produces a lack of sensation.

**Antibodies**
Proteins that specifically stick to foreign material such as bacteria enabling the body to destroy them.

**Antidiuretic hormone**
Hormone controlling the volume of urine passed by the kidney.

**Arteriovenous**
Communication between oxygenated arterial blood and blood of low oxygen content in the veins.

**Bilirubin**
Yellow pigment, increased amounts cause jaundice. Produced when haemoglobin is broken down in the liver.

**Biopsy**
Removal of small amount of body tissue for diagnostic reasons.

**Buprenorphine**
The chemical name for Temgesic which is a powerful pain killer taken under the tongue with less risk of dependency (addiction) than morphine.

**Caesarean section**
Delivery of a baby by abdominal operation.
**Cataracts**
Clouding in the lens of the eye causing blindness that can be corrected by surgery.
**Cerebrovascular**
Relating to the blood system of the brain.
**Chelator**
Strong binding of, for example, iron, enabling it to be removed from the body.
**Chlorpromazine**
A powerful tranquillizer that increases the effectiveness of strong pain killers.
**Cholecystitis**
Inflammation and infection of the gall bladder.
**Chorionic villus sampling**
Removal of a small amount of tissue through the neck of the womb very early in pregnancy enabling diagnosis to be made on the baby.
**Chronic renal failure**
Irreversible and continuous kidney failure.
**Cirrhosis**
Scarring of the liver following damage to the liver from infection, alcohol or iron overload.
**Creatinine**
A break-down product of the body passed out by the kidneys.
**Cyanate**
A chemical that can reduce the sickling of sickle cells in the blood but which also has unacceptable side effects.
**Cyproterone acetate**
A hormone that counteracts some of the effects of male hormone such as testosterone.
**Cystic fibrosis**
An inherited condition causing damage to the lungs and pancreas.
**Cytotoxic**
Drugs or radiation that kill cells as a deliberate effect of treatment.
**Deep vein thrombosis**
Blood clots in the veins of the legs, thighs and pelvis.

**Depo-Provera**
A hormone that can suppress ovulation and so act as a contraceptive.
**Desferrioxamine**
A drug that binds iron enabling it to be passed out by the kidneys.
**Diazepam**
A tranquillizer usually known as Valium.
**Dihydrocodeine**
A moderately powerful pain killer useful for more chronic pain. Derived from codeine.
**Eclampsia**
High blood pressure, swelling of the legs and loss of protein in the urine occurring in late pregnancy.
**Endocrine glands**
Glands that produce hormones that travel through the blood and have their effect in other tissues of the body, e.g. thyroid, pituitary.
**Enuresis**
Urine incontinence, as in bedwetting.
**Epidural**
Anaesthetics given into the spinal column that produce pain relief and loss of sensation in the lower part of the body without affecting the patient's awareness. Used in childbirth.
**Epileptic**
Brain disorder marked by convulsive fits or seizures.
**Erythropoietin**
A hormone produced by the kidney that stimulates the bone marrow to produce red cells and haemoglobin.
**Euphoriant**
Drug which causes an exaggerated sense of well-being.
**Falciparum malaria**
The most serious and dangerous form of malaria, endemic in parts of Africa, India and Far East.
**Ferritin**
Substance for storing iron in the liver and muscles prior to use.
**Folic acid**
A vitamin required for the normal production of healthy red cells.

**Genetic engineering**
Techniques aimed at treating disease by changing the genetic make-up of the individual.
**Glomerular filtration rate**
Volume of fluid that is filtered by the kidneys in one hour.
**Glomerulus**
The part of the kidney that filters the blood that produces urine.
**Haematocrit**
Ratio of red cells to fluid by volume in the blood.
**Haematologist**
A doctor specializing in the management and diagnosis of blood disorders.
**Haematuria**
Passing of blood in the urine.
**Haemoglobin**
Constituent of red blood cells containing a complex of iron and protein capable of binding with oxygen. Used to transport oxygen in the bloodstream. It is responsible for the red colour of blood.
**Haemolysis**
Increased destruction of red blood cells.
**Haemolytic anaemia**
Increased destruction of red cells such that the normal level of haemoglobin falls and the patient is anaemic.
**Haemophilia**
Inherited bleeding tendency caused by deficiency of a blood clotting factor.
**Heparin**
Drug that can be used to prevent clotting of the blood both in patients and in the laboratory.
**Hepatitis**
Inflammation of the liver usually caused by viruses.
**Homozygous**
Having the same gene occurring on both chromosomes. A homozygous sickle cell carrier has two sickle haemoglobin genes.
**Hormone**
Substance produced by endocrine glands that is transported by the blood to have its effect in other tissues.

**Human Immunodeficiency Virus**
The virus which causes AIDS (Acquired Immunodeficiency Syndrome).
**Hydroxyurea**
A drug that interferes with cell function and can produce a cytotoxic effect that is short lived. Used in cancer and leukaemia treatment.
**Ibuprofen**
A drug useful for moderate pain that can reduce inflammation.
**Immunity**
Resistance to infection.
**Impotence**
Inability to have erections of the penis and perform the sexual act.
**Indomethacin**
A potent drug for reducing inflammation. Used in treatment of arthritis.
**Infarct**
Dead area of tissue caused by interruption to its blood supply.
**Intramuscular**
Injection into the substance of the muscle.
**Jaundice**
Increased bilirubin causing yellow colour of the skin and eyes.
**Leukaemia**
Disease characterized by increased production of white blood cells.
**Lymph gland**
Small organs such as the tonsils that are responsible for co-ordinating responses to infection.
**Magnetic Resonance Imaging**
A sophisticated form of computerized imaging that can produce three-dimensional pictures of the body's interior.
**Malaria**
Infection caused by a parasite transmitted by a type of mosquito. Causes periodic attacks of shivering, headaches, vomiting, fever and sweating.
**Maxolon**
An anti-emetic drug – i.e. prevents vomiting.
**Medroxyprogesterone acetate**
The active ingredient in Depo-Provera.

**Medulla**
The innermost part of the kidney responsible for concentrating urine.
**Meningococcus**
A bacterium that can cause meningitis.
**Metoclopromide**
An anti-sickness drug. The active ingredient in Maxolon.
**Morphine**
A very potent pain killer, derived from opium.
**Myocardial infarction**
Heart attack resulting from destruction of heart muscle.
**Neuropathy**
Damage to nerves in the arms or legs leading to loss of sensation and/or muscle weakness.
**Nitrous oxide**
Laughing gas, can be used as a pain killer and anaesthetic.
**Non steroidal anti-inflammatory drugs (NSAIDs)**
Drugs that reduce inflammation such as Aspirin, Ibuprofen, Indomethacin. Used in treatment of arthritis and as pain killers.
**Osmolality**
Salt concentration in urine or blood.
**Osteomyelitis**
Infection of bone.
**Oxygen tension**
Amount of oxygen dissolved in the blood.
**Papillae**
Small projections of the medulla of the kidney.
**Penicillin**
Widely used antibiotic.
**Pethidine**
A powerful pain killer.
**Phenylketonuria**
An inherited condition leading to mental deficiency caused by an excess of phenylketones in the blood.
**Pneumococcus**
A bacterium that can cause pneumonia and meningitis.

**Polymers**
A specific aggregation of proteins or other molecules.
**Priapsim**
Sustained erection of the penis without sexual desire. Usually extremely painful.
**Prochlorperazine**
An anti-sickness drug.
**Prodromal**
A minor illness or sensation that suggests to the patient or to doctors that a more serious illness such as sickle cell crisis is about to occur.
**Progesterone**
A female hormone used as part of a contraceptive pill. Natural progesterone is involved in menstruation and pregnancy.
**Prosthetic**
Artificial limb or apparatus.
**Pulmonary embolism**
A blood clot from a deep vein thrombosis breaking off and lodging in the lung. Can cause severe pain, breathlessness and even death.
**Radiograph**
X-ray picture.
**Rehydration**
Replacement of lost fluid or water.
**Rhesus**
Blood types. Individuals are either rhesus positive or rhesus negative.
**Salmonella**
A bacterium that can cause food poisoning but also serious infections including osteomyelitis.
**Serum**
Clear straw-coloured liquid left after blood is allowed to clot.
**Sicklecrit**
Percentage of haemoglobin S in the blood as a proportion of the haematocrit.
**Sickling**
Deformation of red cells caused by polymerization of haemoglobins.

**Spermatogenesis**
Production of sperm in the testes.
**Spherocytosis**
Disorder of red blood cell production. Can cause haemolytic anaemia.
**Stematil**
Anti-sickness drug and tranquillizer, the active ingredient which is Prochlorperazine.
**Subcutaneous**
An injection just under the skin.
**Sublingual**
Placing a drug under the tongue to allow absorption.
**Temgesic**
*See* Buprenorphine.
**Thrombosis**
Clotting of blood in blood vessels in the body.
**Thyroid**
Gland situated in the neck responsible for growth, development and metabolism.
**Toxicity**
An adverse effect expected or otherwise of a drug, toxin or micro-organism.
**Transcutaneous nerve stimulants (TENS)**
Method of easing pain by stimulation of nerves with an electric current placed on the skin.
**Transfusion**
Giving of blood and other fluids into a vein.
**Tubule**
Part of the kidney medulla responsible for concentrating urine.
**Ulcer**
A breakdown in the surface of the skin, mouth or gut.
**Ultrasound**
Use of high frequency sound waves as in radar to detect abnormalities within the body. Particularly useful in pregnancy where X-rays would harm the fetus.
**Urea**
A chemical excreted by the kidney.

**Valium**

*See* Diazepam.

**Varicose veins**

Enlarged veins due to non-functioning valves. Most common in the legs where blood collects due to gravity.

# Figures and Tables

## FIGURES



## TABLES

ONE

# What is Sickle Cell Disease?

## ORIGINS

Sickle cell disease is a condition which is strongly associated with black people in the minds of the medical profession and the public. But although sickle cell disease has its highest incidence amongst black people it also affects other races. It has its origins among those peoples from parts of the world where malaria, and particularly falciparum malaria, is or was endemic. For this reason sickle cell disease is found in people of African origin, particularly from states in West Africa and sub-Saharan Africa, north of the Zambesi river. It is also found, but less commonly, among the peoples surrounding the Mediterranean, in particular Greece, Cyprus and the Middle East. There are also populations that are affected in India. In order to understand sickle cell disease it is important to appreciate how it came about and why it has become common in certain populations.

## MALARIA

Sickle cell disease developed as a 'by-product' of human defence mechanisms against malaria. The most severe form of malaria, falciparum malaria, leads to a very high death rate in young infants. This is particularly a problem between the time immediately after birth, when they are protected by immunity from the mother, and the time when they are old enough to acquire their own immunity. This period is between about three months and one year of age. Malaria is a parasite which lives within the red blood cells and feeds off the protein that is contained within those red cells, haemoglobin.

Haemoglobin is the molecule which is responsible for transferring oxygen from the lungs, where oxygen is breathed in, to the tissues which use the oxygen to provide energy for cellular functions and activities. In the lungs, where the blood vessels are large, the red cells have no trouble passing through them; but when they reach the tissues the blood vessels become very small and red cells have to be able to squeeze through small openings to deliver their oxygen. The blood vessels become larger again as the blood returns to the lung. The malarial parasites enter the blood stream following the bite of a mosquito. They then penetrate red blood cells by attaching to the outside membrane or envelope of the red cell and gaining entry. Once within the red cell they use the haemoglobin as a source of energy and multiply within it. When the parasites have multiplied so much that they have filled up the red cell it bursts, releasing them into the blood. Each new young parasite enters a single red cell once again. This process perpetuates the disease. As the cells burst and release the parasites into the blood the patient feels ill and develops a fever. In severe forms of falciparum malaria there are so many parasites in the red cells that they become unable to pass through the narrow gaps in the smallest blood vessels and block up tissues, including the brain, leading to death.

Over the centuries human beings have developed a number of strategies to prevent malaria becoming serious and potentially lethal. Some of these modifications affect the red cell membrane to prevent the parasite getting in. But the most common are changes in the type of haemoglobin within the red cell which slow down the ability of the parasite to multiply. One of the most effective ways of preventing the parasite from multiplying is to have sickle haemoglobin or haemoglobin S (Hb S).

The main part of the haemoglobin that we inherit from our parents is present on two genes called beta globin genes. One of these genes is received from each parent. From time to time minor changes or mutations occur in these genes, causing changes in the protein that they produce. A single specific change in the beta globin gene will lead to sickle haemoglobin (haemoglobin S) being produced, instead of the usual haemoglobin A. The first people to have this change would have had sickle haemoglobin produced by only one of their beta globin genes. The other one would have been producing haemoglobin A. Their haemoglobin content in the blood would therefore have consisted of approximately equal quantities of haemoglobin A and haemoglobin S. These individuals are now known as having sickle cell trait or being carriers of sickle cell haemoglobin.

It is difficult for the falciparum malaria parasite to multiply in red cells that contain sickle haemoglobin. This is because the sickle haemoglobin, when it has given up its oxygen, can stick together to form crystalline groupings of haemoglobin, known as polymers. These polymers also distort the red cells into bizarre, 'sickle' shapes, hence the name of the condition (Fig. 1). The presence of these crystalline polymers within the red cells inhibits the growth of the malarial parasite. This prevents the parasite infecting enough red cells for malarial parasites to build up in the tissue of the brain. Therefore, although such individuals can still catch malaria and may become quite ill with it, they are protected from the most

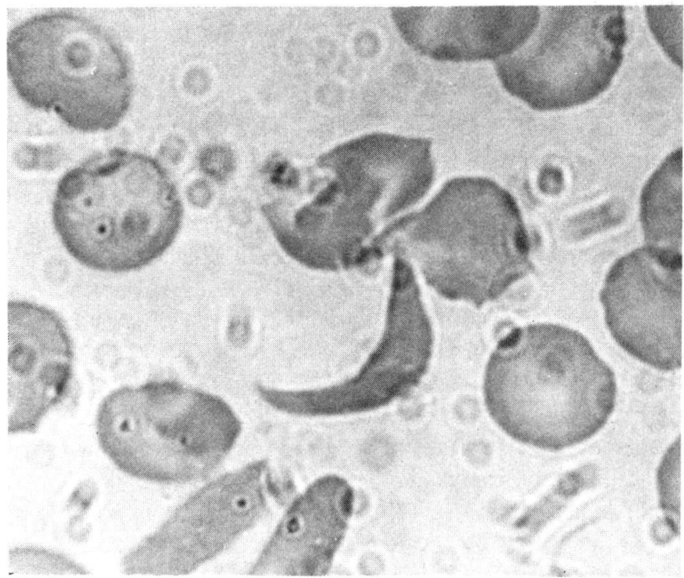

**Fig. 1** Micrograph of sickle cells in blood

severe effects. This benefit has been shown to be most important in the first year of life before the body's natural immunity through antibodies takes over.

## INHERITANCE

Because of this relative resistance to dying from malaria early in life, individuals who have sickle cell trait would have become more likely to survive into adulthood and to pass on their sickle haemoglobin gene to their children. Therefore those families which carried the sickle haemoglobin gene would have become more common, and prospered. Eventually, individuals who were both sickle cell trait, and therefore carried the haemoglobin S gene, would have children. In such a partnership, if both parents carry the sickle haemoglobin gene, there is a one in four chance that any one child will receive the sickle haemoglobin gene from one parent and also from the other. This is how two healthy parents, who each have one haemoglobin S gene, can produce a child who, because it has two haemoglobin S genes, suffers from sickle cell disease. A person with two haemoglobin S genes has virtually only sickle haemoglobin in his/her red blood cells, and produces so much crystalline polymer within the red blood cells that the cells become permanently stiff and damaged as they pass through the circulation. The advantages of resistance to malaria are therefore lost because of the complications produced by these stiff red cells which lead to the condition known as sickle cell disease. Thus, sickle cell disease is, in many respects, a by-product of human's strategies to avoid succumbing to falciparum malaria. This is why sickle cell disease is most common in Kenya and parts of West Africa where falciparum malaria is most common.

It is important for couples in whom one or both has sickle cell trait, or another haemoglobin disorder, to know the possible types of disorder that could affect their children. One of the two beta haemoglobin genes is passed on to each child, but *which* one is a random event. Therefore, each child of a parent who has sickle cell trait has a 50:50 chance of getting the Hb S gene rather than the

Hb A one. Because the same applies to the other parent, there are four possible combinations (Fig. 2).

So, *on average*, two children will have sickle cell trait (A/S), one will have only haemoglobin A (A/A) and one will have sickle cell disease (S/S) – known as homozygous sickle cell disease. But every child has the same chance, one in four, of having the S/S, so previous children do not help predict the haemoglobin type of the next child. Table 1 shows some important haemoglobin types that can interact between parents.

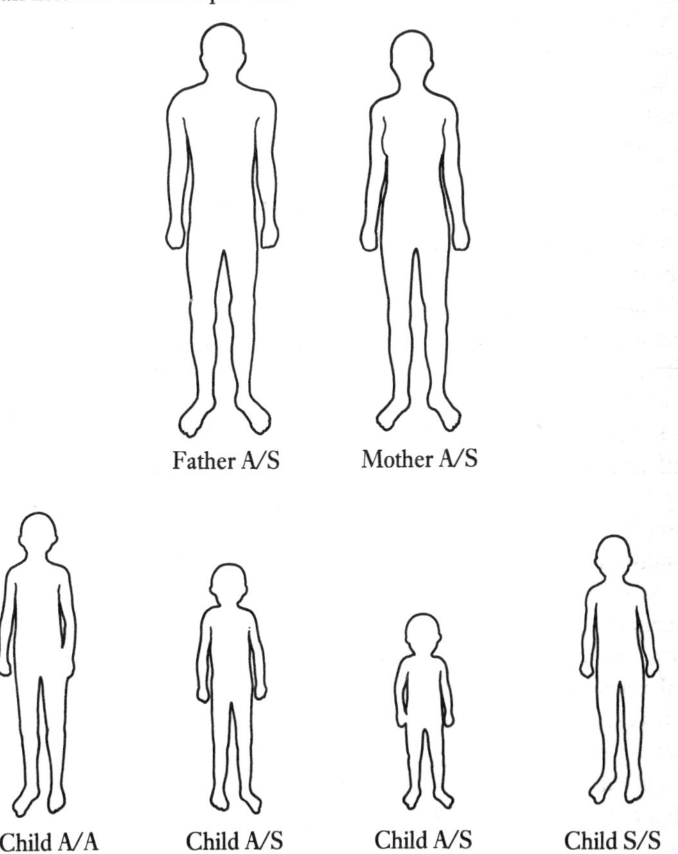


**Fig. 2** Inheritance of sickle haemoglobin

**Table 1** Combinations of haemoglobin types

1 *Sickle cell trait and haemoglobin A only*

| | 1 | | 2 | |
|---|---|---|---|---|
| Parents | Sickle cell trait | | Haemoglobin A | |
| Haemoglobin type | A/S | | A/A | |
| Children | A/A | A/S | A/S | A/A |

Each child has a 50:50 chance of having haemoglobin A only or of having sickle cell trait, because all children get Hb A from parent 2, and have a 50:50 chance of getting Hb S from parent 1.

2 *Homozygous SS disease and haemoglobin A only*

| | 1 | | 2 | |
|---|---|---|---|---|
| Parents | Homozygous SS disease | | Haemoglobin A | |
| Haemoglobin type | S/S | | A/A | |
| Children | A/S | A/S | A/S | A/S |

All children will have sickle cell trait, because parent 1 always passes on Hb S and parent 2 always gives Hb A.

3 *Homozygous SS disease and sickle cell trait*

| | 1 | | 2 | |
|---|---|---|---|---|
| Parents | Homozygous SS disease | | Sickle cell trait | |
| Haemoglobin types | S/S | | A/S | |
| Children | S/S | S/S | A/S | A/S |

All children have a 50:50 chance of having sickle cell disease or sickle cell trait.

4 *Sickle cell trait and haemoglobin C trait*

| | 1 | | 2 | |
|---|---|---|---|---|
| Parents | Sickle cell trait | | Haemoglobin C trait | |
| Haemoglobin types | A/S | | A/C | |
| Children | A/A | S/A | S/C | A/C |

Because both parents have one Hb A gene, there is a 1:4 chance of each child having Hb A only. There is also a 1:4 chance of having Hb C trait or sickle trait *or* Hb S/Hb C disease.

5 *Sickle cell beta° thalassaemia and beta° thalassaemia trait*

| | 1 | | 2 |
|---|---|---|---|
| Parents | Sickle cell/beta° thalassaemia | | Beta° thalassaemia trait |
| Haemoglobin types | S/B° thal | | A/B° thal |
| Children | A/S | S/B° thal | A/B° thal<br>B°thal/B° thal |

There is a 1:4 chance of each of the four possibilities occurring for each child. The two beta° thalassaemia genes combine to give a 1:4 chance of thalassaemia major, a severe anaemia that needs blood transfusions from six months of age.

---

## SPREAD OF SICKLE CELL DISEASE

Sickle cell disease spread to many parts of the world during the colonization of North and South America, mainly through the slave trade. Sickle cell disease is now found in the UK as a result of immigration from the Caribbean and from Africa. Emigration from Greece and Cyprus has also brought some sickle cell disease to Western Europe and Australia, although these populations have more thalassaemia, which is another mechanism for avoiding malarial infections. All this worldwide spread of sickle cell disease took place by the carriers of the sickle cell trait migrating, either forcibly or voluntarily. The disease cannot be acquired in any way other than inheritance.

### Sickle Cell Disease in Africa

Central Africa, from south of the Sahara to north of the Zambesi river, is the area where sickle cell disease is most common. In some parts of West Africa and Kenya, where falciparum malaria has its highest incidence, as many as 30 per cent of the population may be carriers of sickle cell trait and up to 3 per cent of infants born will have sickle cell disease. Before the availability of antibiotics and antimalarials most of these affected children died. Even now, it is thought that the mortality from sickle cell disease in rural areas of

Africa is extremely high in the first year of life, and it is only in the larger cities that children with sickle cell disease have a reasonable chance of survival into adulthood. The exploitation of black Africans in the slave trade led to the spread of sickle cell disease to north and south America and the Caribbean islands. The great majority of the individuals who took the sickle cell gene to the New World would have had sickle cell trait and have been quite healthy. It would have been their children who were at risk of suffering from sickle cell disease. No doubt in the harsh environments of slavery few such sickle cell sufferers would have survived.

## Sickle Cell Disease in America and Britain

In the New World, away from the influence of falciparum malaria, the incidence of the sickle cell haemoglobin gene slowly started to decrease. It has now reached a point where, in North America, it affects approximately 8 per cent of Americans of African descent. A similar percentage of carriers is found in immigrants from the West Indies to the United Kingdom. The natural history of sickle cell disease is probably best understood in Jamaica because of the work of Professor Graham Serjeant and his colleagues. Again the majority of the emigrants to the UK who have carried the sickle cell gene with them would have been healthy carriers, with only a few mildly affected individuals with sickle cell disease being fit enough to emigrate.

Since the main immigration to the United Kingdom took place in the 1950s and 1960s there has been an increasing incidence of sickle cell disease amongst British people of Afro-Caribbean descent throughout the 1970s and into the 1980s. Testing of all new-born babies for sickle cell disease has been undertaken in Birmingham since 1979 and this clearly shows a steady increase in the numbers of babies with sickle cell disease being detected. This increase is in the children of healthy carriers who migrated to the United Kingdom. So, even though the proportion of sickle trait carriers is slowly declining, the numbers in the UK increased significantly following the 1950s' immigration.

There is a general feeling that sickle cell disease in the United

Kingdom is less severe than in Jamaica. Such a supposition is difficult to prove and is perhaps a little surprising given the pleasant climate of Jamaica in contrast to the colder one in the UK. As will be discussed later, exposure to cold and damp tends to make sickle cell crises more likely and it might be expected that symptoms in the UK would be worse. However, the standard of living is higher in the UK and access to medical care more immediate. As in the case of infectious disease it is probably the improving standard of living in terms of sanitation, heating and shelter that leads to the more mild outcome of the disease in Britain.

## Sickle Cell Disease in India

There are two main areas where sickle cell disease occurs in India. One of these is in the highlands of central India, the Veddid area, and the other is in Orissa State. Most of the immigrants to the UK from the Indian subcontinent do not come from these areas and therefore the incidence of sickle cell disease in the Asian population in the UK is quite small. However, there is a possibility that individuals from the Indian subcontinent might have sickle cell disease. Therefore, it is considered by some that such people should be tested for sickle cell disease before anaesthesia and surgery. At the present time however this is not done as a routine in Britain.

## Sickle Cell Disease in the Middle East and the Mediterranean

Sickle cell carriers are rather less frequent in these areas than in Africa or among Afro-Caribbean peoples. However, other abnormal haemoglobins also occur in these groups, in particular beta thalassaemia. Individuals who have a combination of sickle cell trait and beta thalassaemia (sickle cell/beta thalassaemia; see p.7) are therefore not uncommon. Some types of beta thalassaemia lead to the production of small amounts of adult haemoglobin A and these individuals have a mild form of sickle cell disease known as sickle cell/beta$^{+}$ thalassaemia. However, those people who have no haemoglobin A at all (sickle cell/beta$^{\circ}$ thalassaemia) have sickle cell disease that is as severe as the homozygous SS form. Parts of Saudi Arabia and Jordan have a particular type of sickle cell disease in which a high level of fetal haemoglobin is characteristic. In these people perhaps 80 per cent of the blood haemoglobin is sickle haemoglobin and 20 per cent is haemoglobin F. This leads to quite a good compromise since the presence of the sickle haemoglobin will make them produce good resistance to falciparum malaria but the high level of fetal haemoglobin prevents significant sickling.

The distribution of the fetal haemoglobin within the red cells is important in these cases. If every single red blood cell contains 20 per cent of fetal haemoglobin and 80 per cent sickle then sickling will be prevented. However if 80 per cent of the red cells contain sickle haemoglobin and 20 per cent of the red cells contain fetal haemoglobin then sickling will be reduced only marginally. This point will be considered further in the section on blood transfusion where it is of particular relevance.

## PAINFUL CRISES AND 'SICKLING'

As we have seen, sickle cell disease is a condition caused by the presence in red blood cells of the sickle haemoglobin, haemoglobin S (Hb S). Sickle haemoglobin is different from the usual haemoglobin (haemoglobin A) in that when it gives up its oxygen in the tissues the Hb S molecules stick together in rigid 'crystals', causing the red blood cells to become deformed and stiff when they are in an area of low oxygen. These stiff red cells can then block small blood vessels leading to the death of a small piece of tissue and causing very severe pain. These episodes of pain are called painful crises. These are dealt with in detail in Chapter 3. The stiff deformed red cells can initially recover their soft shape when they return to the lungs and are re-oxygenated but after a number of cycles the membrane envelope of the cell becomes irreparably damaged and the cells become irreversibly sickled cells (ISCs). These ISCs survive in the circulation for only a couple of weeks instead of the normal red cell life of 120 days. This more rapid destruction of red cells in sickle cell disease is called haemolysis.

The bone marrow tries to keep up with the increased destruction by making more red cells but is only partly successful. Most patients with sickle cell disease are also anaemic because of this inadequate response by the bone marrow to the haemolysis. This type of anaemia is called haemolytic anaemia. One of the other properties of sickle haemoglobin is that it can give up more oxygen to the tissues than normal haemoglobin. This means that even though the anaemia is quite severe the tissues of the body still receive sufficient oxygen, until the time a painful crisis occurs. Symptoms of anaemia are therefore quite unusual in sufferers from sickle cell disease, even though they have low oxygen in their blood.

TWO

# The Sickle Cell Carrier (Sickle Cell Trait)

Carriers of sickle cell disease are healthy people who have a normal blood count, are not anaemic and have a normal life expectancy. They are as capable as anyone of training as athletes and are represented in normal numbers among American football players. Individuals with sickle cell trait competed successfully at altitude in the Mexico Olympic Games. Medical opinion is that individuals who are carriers of sickle haemoglobin have no symptoms whatever referable to it other than occasional problems of the urinary tract. This means they do not get painful sickle crises, and any aches and pains that they suffer from should not be attributed to their sickle cell carrier state. This view is not held by all members of the sickle cell community, however, and can lead to misunderstandings. It must be said that there do not appear to be any in-depth studies with good controls that have looked at whether individuals with sickle cell trait do get more aches and pains in the bones or muscles than similar individuals who have only haemoglobin A.

The discovery that a person is a carrier for sickle cell haemoglobin should not lead to any major consequences regarding life insurance or their job. There are only a very few occupations from which they are excluded, such as working in submarines and as airforce fighter pilots. These exclusions are based on occasional reports of possible sickle crises occurring in individuals with sickle cell trait who were exposed to extremely low oxygen levels. Individuals with sickle trait are accepted as members of aircrew other than on the flight deck.

## Problems of Having the Sickle Cell Trait

Ordinarily red blood cells in a sickle cell carrier will each have about 60 per cent haemoglobin A and 40 per cent haemoglobin S. Even though there is so much HbA present, the HbS can still form polymers when there is very little oxygen. This means that it is possible for the red cells in sickle trait blood to become sickled, but only under the most extreme circumstances. The most frequent place for this to occur is in part of the kidney where the salt concentration becomes extremely high causing the red cells to dry out. Under these conditions red cell sickling can occur and results in damage to that part of the kidney. This never leads to kidney failure but can cause bleeding into the urine and reduction in the ability of the kidney to concentrate urine properly. This means that the individual with sickle cell trait may pass more urine than a person with normal haemoglobin and this can lead to problems with bed wetting (enuresis). Also women with sickle cell trait when pregnant suffer from more urinary tract infections than those with only haemoglobin A. Under very extreme conditions of very low oxygen tension there have been occasional reports of sickle crises occurring in people with sickle cell trait. Damage to the spleen caused by loss of blood (infarcts) have also been reported. For these reasons it is important that the presence of sickle cell trait is known about before operations so that good oxygenation of the patient can be maintained.

Of course, the other major consideration of someone with sickle cell trait is that they are capable of passing it on to their children. Moreover, if their partner is also a carrier, or has sickle cell disease or beta thalassaemia, there is a significant risk that some of their children will have a form of sickle cell disease. For this reason it is important that people should know whether or not they are carriers of sickle cell trait. It is possible to test for this at birth or in early childhood but the main reason for testing so early is to detect sufferers of sickle cell disease. At present there is no known benefit of informing individuals that they have sickle cell trait at a very early age but certainly individuals should be informed during adolescence before they become sexually active. However, at the present time in the UK there are no facilities or plans to develop screening and counselling services for older school age children.

Once an individual is aware that he or she has sickle cell trait then this is something that needs to be considered when thinking of having a family. It is unlikely that such information would influence their choice of partner although, in some populations, people who carry beta thalassaemia trait do consider this. It would seem to be of importance that a couple should know whether they are at risk of having children with sickle cell disease so that they may decide what they wish to do about it. Further consideration of antenatal diagnosis and counselling regarding the likelihood of children having sickle cell disease is considered in Chapter 7.

The term 'having sickle' is sometimes used for individuals who have the sickle cell trait. This is a confusing term since it can often be taken to include sickle cell disease sufferers. It is of utmost importance to clarify both in the individual's mind and also in any health professional whom they consult whether they have sickle cell disease or are healthy carriers of the trait. It would be much better if the term healthy carrier could be substituted for the more imprecise term.

## Testing for Sickle Cell Haemoglobin

The rights and wrongs of testing for sickle cell disease and sickle cell carriers have been the cause of much discussion over the past twenty years. In the past few years in the UK there has been a feeling within the black community that individuals have a right to know whether they are carriers of sickle haemoglobin or not. Anyone who has been informed about sickle cell disease and its consequences, and who then decides that they would like to know whether they are a sickle cell carrier, should be able to have a test. However, there have been occasions, particularly in the United States, where programmes of testing individuals have been undertaken, when unexpected, unwelcome and unacceptable outcomes have resulted. For this reason it is important that any facilities offering testing to people or communities should be carefully controlled and monitored so that the effects of the testing are beneficial and not harmful.

*Mass Screening*

The use of mass screening commenced in the United States during the Presidency of Richard Nixon. Large networks of sickle cell centres were set up and community screening programmes were established. In some States it even became compulsory to be tested if you were black. Unfortunately these programmes were set up with inadequate support in terms of education, counselling and information to the community at large. This resulted in many healthy individuals with sickle cell trait being denied life insurance and having additional problems with employment. These programmes also led to some black consciousness groups becoming very concerned that the testing programmes were part of systematic discrimination against black people. For this reason community testing fell into disrepute. Certainly as carried out at that time this was the deserved result.

One result, however, was that it made doctors in the UK very cautious about introducing testing programmes for the community. In general such schemes have been developed in the UK following pressure from the community itself. This has led to much criticism of the health services for dragging their feet and failing to provide adequately for testing. This sequence of events has at least had the advantage that testing services have been set up at the request of the community and often after much canvassing. This has meant that such programmes have had the support of the local community and are therefore much more likely to be successsful and used.

*Voluntary Testing*

The mass screening of whole populations that was carried out in the late 1960s/early 1970s has given way to the view that testing should be freely and readily available but on a voluntary basis for those who wish to take advantage of it. In addition it has become accepted that testing should be preceded by an educational session in which details of sickle cell disease and the significance and relevance of having sickle cell trait are discussed. For those individuals who are found to have only normal haemoglobin this pre-test interview is the only one offered unless they specifically request further discussion. In Birmingham only those who have a positive test are recalled for further talks with the Sickle Cell Counsellor. A few months after the test at the post-test educational session a further appointment is arranged for those who wish to be seen again. This gives an opportunity to check that the information given at the previous interviews has been retained. In particular the method of inheritance of sickle cell disease is stressed and the fact that sickle cell carriers are healthy. In this way it is hoped to minimize any negative psychological effects on individuals who are positive for sickle cell trait. We can also be certain that they understand its significance in the way in which it can be passed on to their children.

*Sickle Haemoglobin Testing in Hospital*

Testing of people in hospital is carried out as a routine. All people of Afro-Caribbean origin are tested for sickle cell disease if they are likely to require a general anaesthetic. This is because general anaesthetics are hazardous to individuals with sickle cell disease if precautions are not taken. Detailed guidelines for testing have been prepared by the British Society for Haematology. These also recommend testing individuals from the Mediterranean and the Asian subcontinent. In practice most hospitals do not carry out this advice at the present time because of the low incidence of sickle cell disease in these other groups.

It is possible for individuals with sickle cell disease to be diagnosed late in life prior to or during anaesthetics and the lack of a preceding history is no guarantee that the individual may not have a milder form of sickle cell disease which may nevertheless be a major problem under anaesthetic.

Obviously most people who have been tested will be clear of the sickle cell haemoglobin but about 8 per cent will be found to be carriers. At the present time it is unusual for any formal counselling or discussion to take place before testing individuals in hospital for sickle cell carrier status. However, following the test the result should be communicated to the patient. Obviously if they are found to have sickle cell disease this will be discussed with them in detail by the doctors caring for the patient and the blood specialist (haematologist). If found to be carriers of sickle haemoglobin they will be given a card which confirms the haemoglobin status and also an explanatory leaflet. Both the card and the leaflet are produced by the Department of Health. The patient's General Practitioner will also be informed. In Birmingham individuals who are tested positive are offered the services of the Sickle Cell Service for further advice. Individuals who test for normal haemoglobin A also receive a card and an explanatory leaflet, although this is thought to be unnecessary by many haematologists.

*Pregnant Women*

In most hospitals pregnant women who are apparently of Afro-Caribbean ethnic origin are tested but a recent study from Cardiff showed that this leads to a significant number of women being missed. In hospitals where greater than 10 per cent of women are likely to be of Afro-Caribbean origin it is considered better to test all pregnant women not only for sickle cell carriers status but also for beta thalassaemia trait.

Pregnant women who have a positive test for sickle cell trait will be informed in a similar manner to the individuals who are tested positive in the general hospital. However, they should also be offered testing of their partner which will make it possible to detect those pregnancies which are at risk of having a child affected by sickle cell disease. Such a system has two advantages. First, it enables counselling to begin at an early stage before the child is born to prepare the parents for the possible birth of a child with sickle cell disease. Obviously this is a very difficult and emotional time for parents particularly if it is their first child. This counselling needs considerable resources and expertise. Since most hospitals would not have very many at-risk pregnancies in a year it is probably best if such counselling is managed by a team of a specific Consultant Obstetrician and Haematologist and also a specific Counsellor. The second advantage of early identification of at-risk pregnancies is that couples may wish to consider antenatal diagnosis and selective abortion of an affected fetus. At the present time few couples wish to consider this option but it is important that couples should have the information available so that they can make their own decisions about their pregnancy.

Testing of the unborn fetus can also be carried out. At the present time this would only be done if the couple had already decided to terminate an affected pregnancy. There are those who feel this should be offered to couples as part of their decision-making process, however. There is a risk of spontaneous abortion following the testing so all the issues must be placed before the couple to enable them to decide. Testing will normally be by amniocentesis at 16 weeks of pregnancy but earlier testing using chorionic villus sampling (CVS) and new DNA diagnostic techniques may be available soon.

*New-born Babies*

The testing of new-born babies is another area of some controversy. As for testing pregnant women it is probably inefficient to simply test those babies that are considered to be from at-risk ethnic groups. Unless the likely incidence of sickle cell disease is very small in an area it is probably better to test all new-born babies. This can be done as part of the testing for phenylketonuria and hypothyroidism that already takes place throughout the UK. Laboratory testing can be automated and is now very accurate. Because of the presence of fetal haemoglobin at birth, babies are quite healthy at that time but it is possible to detect the absence of normal haemoglobin A and the presence of only haemoglobin S in addition to the fetal haemoglobin. Clearly any baby found to have sickle cell disease should be recalled to the clinic, retested to confirm the diagnosis and the parents informed and counselled. Such a procedure should greatly reduce the levels of anxiety of the parents if carried out effectively. An undiagnosed child with sickle cell disease will become ill at some point in the first year or so of life. Occasionally sickle cell disease can go undiagnosed for some time. This causes much anxiety in the parents as symptoms can be worrying.

There is now evidence emerging to show that diagnosis at birth can prevent admissions to hospital and perhaps even death. Parents may be made aware from an early stage of what problems their child may face. This can make them vigilant for specific problems like painful crisis, hand–foot syndrome and serious infections.

The main dilemma regarding screening of the new-born has been what to do with those babies that have been found to have sickle cell trait rather than sickle cell disease. To adopt a policy of informing parents that their child was a carrier of sickle trait would require a major investment in counselling facilities to ensure that such children did not suffer from being thought to have a disease or illness. Furthermore, it would still be important to reinforce the information to the child particularly when the child reached adolescence and entered the child-bearing years. At the present time it is not policy to inform parents that their child is a carrier for sickle cell haemoglobin. There are many ethical arguments for and against disclosure of the information and possible courses of action need to be discussed in detail both among the health care professions and also among the communities at risk of sickle cell disease.

## SUMMARY

Individuals who are carriers for the sickle cell trait are healthy, have a normal life expectancy and are free to pursue a normal life. They may have increased problems with their kidneys with occasional problems of passing blood in the urine or water infections. It is important that people know whether or not they are carriers of sickle cell trait so that they can decide for themselves what they would like to do if and when they are at risk of having a child with sickle cell disease.

THREE
# Sickle Cell Crises

There are three main types of sickle cell crises.

1 Painful crisis (including life-threatening complications such as chest syndrome and girdle syndrome)
2 Anaemic crisis
3 Sequestration crisis

## PAINFUL CRISIS

The painful crisis is the most common and frequent complication affecting individuals with sickle cell disease. It particularly affects people who have homozygous SS disease and sickle cell beta thalassaemia (see p.7). It is less common in individuals with haemoglobin S/haemoglobin C disease. There is an enormous variation between patients and the number of painful crises they have each year. The average number is three. This can vary from individuals having six, seven or eight crises a year to having none at all. Crises last on average about seven days but can be anything from two or three days to three or four weeks. They often come out of the blue and are extremely disruptive to education, employment and life in general. Severe crises particularly when they involve the lungs (chest syndrome) or the liver and abdomen (girdle syndrome) can be life threatening. The typical painful crisis starts with some warning to the patient. About a third of sickle cell patients experience what is called a *prodromal phase* to their crisis. This prodromal phase warns the patient that a crisis is about to occur but it is often difficult for the patient to describe. This continues until the pain develops, most commonly in the limbs but often in the back and sometimes in the chest. The pain is deep seated and very severe and comes from the bones. At this stage the patient can often control the pain with powerful pain killers taken by mouth and by drinking large amounts of fluid each day (6 pints or about 3 litres). If they can go to bed, rest and keep warm it may be possible for them to manage their pain at home. Probably the majority of crises are managed by the patient at home in this way and never come to the attention of hospital doctors. Those crises that continue and become severe are the ones that are most commonly seen in hospital. The patient is usually in severe pain and, by the time they arrive in hospital, are often very dehydrated. This dehydration is a major problem since it makes the blood more viscous, encourages sickling of red cells, and therefore makes the crisis worse. The worse the crisis gets the more dehydrated the patient becomes and so on. Dehydration is difficult to control in sickle cell patients because of the damage to the kidneys which means that urine output is not shut down and the urine more concentrated (see Chapter 4). Therefore, even when the patient is quite dry they continue to produce significant quantities of urine. On admission to hospital any other possible causes of the pain must be excluded since it is of course possible for sickle cell patients to suffer from appendicitis, gall stones and arthritis just as any other person can. They will then receive pain relief either by mouth or more usually by injection. This aspect will be considered in more detail in Chapter 4. Together with the pain relief, intravenous fluids will almost always be given although some patients who can manage to drink may prefer to do so. At least 3–4 litres of fluid a day will be required and often patients with severe crises who are very dry need 6 litres of fluid in the first day to catch up with their fluid balance. Most patients with a painful crisis do not have infections as a predisposing cause but it is important for doctors to look for these since occasionally urinary tract infections or chest infections are uncovered.

Patients often develop a temperature either at the time of admission or soon after and most patients with a painful crisis receive some form of antibiotic. This is not necessary to the management of the painful crisis itself, but ensures that there is no complicating infection. Although patients are suffering a lack of oxygen in their blood supply, oxygen is not thought to help in the uncomplicated painful crisis, but it is used if there is any involvement of the lungs. The reason that oxygen is not effective is that since the blood supply is interrupted to the area of tissue from which the pain is coming, oxygen inhaled by mouth will not get to that area in any case. Trials of inhaling oxygen under very high pressure have likewise not been beneficial. Most patients will be able to stop receiving the intramuscular or intravenous pain killing injections after about three or four days and can be switched to tablets for a further two to three days before stopping pain killing tablets altogether. The usual period for remaining in hospital is about seven days.

## Chest Syndrome

About 5–10 per cent of patients with a painful crisis develop abnormalities on the chest radiograph two or three days after admission. This is thought to reflect sickling occurring within the lungs. Chest infection may be present and for this reason the term chest syndrome has been coined. Chest syndrome is a most serious complication of sickle cell crisis and warrants urgent treatment. All patients with a moderately severe painful crisis should have a chest radiograph taken on the second or third day of their admission unless they are already clearly improving. This is because the chest radiograph taken on admission to hospital is usually clear even in cases that ultimately develop chest syndrome. The presence of patchy shadowing on the radiograph should lead to the patient having a blood sample taken from an artery to look for the blood gas levels of oxygen, carbon dioxide and pH. This will confirm whether the lungs are performing normally or adequately. If they are not the patient will be started on oxygen and monitored very closely. If there is any sign of deterioration or if the oxygenation of the blood is unsatisfactory the patient will be prepared for an emergency exchange blood transfusion. This should be carried out as described in Chapter 6. Chest syndrome is the most common cause of death from sickle cell disease in adulthood and should be treated very promptly.

## ANAEMIC CRISES

Anaemic crises are quite uncommon in sickle cell disease and are usually seen in childhood. However, they can occasionally occur in adults. There are two types, one in which the bone marrow suddenly stops producing red blood cells, usually because of an infection of parvovirus. The second type is associated with massive enlargement of the spleen which is filled with blood. Because the blood is sequestered, i.e. trapped in the spleen, these crises are also called sequestration crises.

### Classic Anaemic Crisis

This develops over a few days and is usually preceded by an illness. This may take the form of a virus infection with a mild fever, some shivering and the child may be off his or her food. When children recover from the virus infection they then become lethargic and pale. They may become so lethargic that they cannot get up and become short of breath on the most minimal exertion. When they attend hospital the haemoglobin may be found to be incredibly low – somewhere between 2 and 4 g/dl as opposed to a normal level of 6 to 9 g/dl in the steady state. The other elements of the blood, the white cells and platelets, are normal. The patient requires blood transfusion to improve the haemoglobin and make them feel better and recovery always takes place within a week or two. Similar problems are also seen in other diseases where the bone marrow is having to work harder to keep up with a haemolytic anaemia. The cause was unknown until a few years ago. Scientists were testing frozen blood specimens for antibodies to parvovirus and found that many patients with sickle cell disease had such antibodies. They then found that the antibodies then coincided with samples taken from a time when they were suffering from an anaemic crisis. It has now been found conclusively that parvovirus is capable of preventing the bone marrow producing red blood cells for a period of a week or so. In the case of normal individuals who suffer from parvovirus infections this would simply cause the blood haemoglobin to fall by 1 or 2 g/dl which would not be noticed by the individual. This is because normal people only produce about 1 per cent of their whole blood each day therefore stopping for ten days does not make that much difference. However, people with sickle cell disease make 5–10 per cent of their blood every day and therefore stopping for a week means that they will lose 50 per cent of their blood. Since they are already anaemic this is obviously very serious and leads to their profound anaemia and weakness. Fortunately it is a self-limiting condition and gets better providing the patient can receive blood transfusion support for the week or two that the problems lasts. Because it is caused by exposure to a virus and immunity is good each individual will only suffer from one anaemic crisis in his or her life.

## SEQUESTRATION CRISES

These are rare but extremely serious episodes set off by infections. They nearly always occur in young children in the first few years of life. The child will become ill with an infection and then become pale and lethargic very quickly. The spleen enlarges massively so that it can on occasions fill most of the abdomen. Very rarely in children who have had their spleen removed, the sequestration can occur in the liver and it is the liver that becomes very large and full of blood. In its most severe form most of the blood in the body is packed into the spleen and there is very little circulating in the blood to convey oxygen to the tissues. Therefore, the child becomes very unwell and weak. To the doctor the appearance is that of a child who has collapsed and perhaps been bleeding or is in shock. The temptation is for the doctor to set up a drip with salt solutions in it but this can be rapidly fatal to the overworked heart and circulation. It is essential in any child with sickle cell disease who becomes rapidly unwell that splenic sequestration crisis is anticipated and the abdomen felt for the masively enlarged spleen. Once the condition is diagnosed, blood should be sent for cross-matching or, if essential, group O negative blood given. Packed red blood cells only should be infused slowly. These are life saving. Because they can convey oxygen to the tissues immediately they help the problem without further overloading the heart. Giving further fluid is counterproductive and the child could die if given just liquids. The exact cause of the condition is not really known. It is known that the blood supply through the spleen appears to be interrupted and that the red blood cells block blood vessels and sickle within the spleen which just gets bigger and bigger as more and more red cells enter it. Once a child has one attack it is at risk of further attacks and it is essential that the mother and carers of children with sickle cell disease know how to examine for an enlarging spleen so that they can rush the child to hospital should it occur. Once there has been one episode, certainly in the UK, removal of the spleen would be considered to prevent further occurrences.

FOUR

# Other Complications of Sickle Cell Disease

In addition to the crises that can befall individuals with sickle cell disease there are numerous other complications that arise because of the condition. None of these are associated with the healthy sickle cell trait carriers. These complications fall broadly into those problems secondary to the haemolytic anaemia and problems secondary to the sickling: for definitions of these terms see the glossary. In addition a specific complication of sickling within the spleen leads to a reduced ability to fight certain infections.

| A *Haemolysis* | B *Sickling* | C *Infections* |
|---|---|---|
| Gall-stones | Kidney disorders | Pneumococcus |
| Jaundice | Joint damage | Salmonella |
| Leg ulcers | Strokes | |
| | Liver disease | |
| | Splenic atrophy | |
| | (leg ulcers?) | |

## PROBLEMS SECONDARY TO HAEMOLYTIC ANAEMIA

These problems affect sufferers with sickle cell disease in the same way that other sufferers with haemolytic anaemias can be affected. This leads to an increased incidence of gall-stones, jaundice and leg ulcers. These problems are also seen in other types of haemolytic anaemia, such as hereditary spherocytosis and thalassaemia.

## Jaundice

As the damaged sickled red cells are removed from the circulation, mainly in the liver and to a lesser extent the spleen, the haemoglobin within the red cells is released and broken down further to a chemical called bilirubin. This is a yellow colour and is responsible for the jaundice that many sufferers from sickle cell disease demonstrate. Bilirubin circulates in the blood until it reaches the liver where it is converted into salts that make it soluble in water. These salts are excreted through the bile into the gut and also through the kidneys. Of itself the jaundice is completely harmless and does not represent hepatitis or liver disease. The degree to which individuals have jaundice varies greatly. Some sickle cell individuals have quite marked yellowness of their eyes. Because most sufferers of sickle cell disease have black skin they do not look yellow other than the eyes and sometimes the palms of the hands. The yellow colour can wax and wane depending on the health of the person. For instance a painful crisis or an infection, cough or cold may make the jaundice worse and the yellow colour brighter. This represents changes in the ability of the liver to deal with the bilirubin and excrete it. It does not usually represent changes in the rate of red cell breakdown.

## Gall-stones

By the age of thirty-five, 80 per cent or more of individuals with homozygous sickle cell disease will have gall-stones in their gall bladder. These stones are formed for the same reason that the individuals are often jaundiced. The bilirubin passes through the liver and into the gut through bile. Because there is an increased amount of bilirubin the bile is thicker than usual and the flow is slower. The gall bladder is a pouch off the bile duct which usually stores bile and squirts it into the gut at appropriate times during digestion. The bile becomes thicker and thicker and eventually the bilirubin starts to crystallize out in the gall bladder as gall-stones. Gall-stones are not a problem in themselves but do reflect sluggish bile circulation through the bile duct and gall bladder and this can be associated with an increased incidence of infection of the gall bladder (cholecystitis). These bouts of infection cause scarring of the gall bladder wall and pain. Repeated episodes would be a reason for removing the gall bladder. Another reason for removing the gall bladder would be repeated pain due to gall-stones partially blocking the outflow of the bile duct or, more seriously, a gall-stone escaping from the gall bladder and then blocking the bile duct. This is associated with a much greater worsening of the jaundice and also severe pain known as gall-stone colic. Removing the gall bladder of a patient with homozygous sickle cell disease is not a matter to be taken lightly and requires very careful preparation before surgery. There is good evidence that exchange blood transfusion in the week or two before the operation significantly reduces the risks of chest infection and sickle crisis following the surgery. In such situations it is important that the level of sickle haemoglobin is reduced to below about 25 per cent. Clearly an operation requiring exchange transfusion is not to be undertaken without good reason. This would not be considered if an individual simply has gall-stones in their gall bladder. Only if they are causing symptoms may gall bladder removal be considered.

Symptoms that may occur with gall-stones are acute bouts of very severe pain associated with fever which is due to cholecystitis. More common is a grumbly sort of pain in the right upper abdomen usually associated with small gall-stones being passed. It is now very easy to detect gall-stones using ultrasound in which a small probe like a microphone is rubbed over the abdomen. This can locate the gall-stones using echoes. Occasionally it is necessary to use some of the older tests in which dye is swallowed and passed out through the gall-bladder. This shows the stones up on an X-ray film (oral cholecystogram).

## Leg Ulcers

The cause of leg ulcers is unknown but it has been assumed that sickling is an important factor. However, leg ulcers do occur quite commonly in individuals with haemolytic anaemias, such as hereditary spherocytosis and thalassaemia, and therefore it is more likely to be a combination of effects (see Fig. 3). Certainly the pressure on

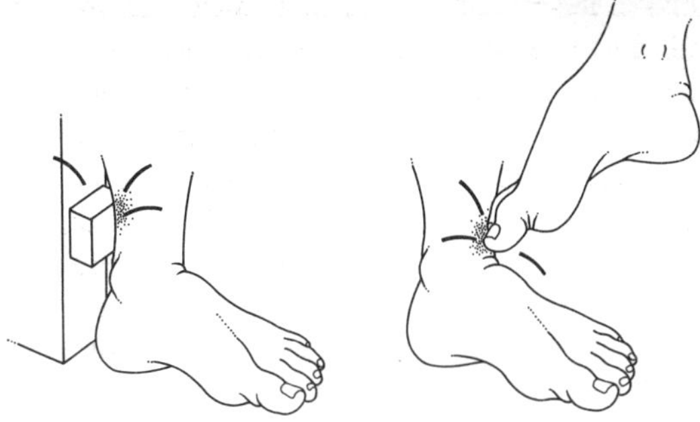

*1 Injury* Minor knocks and kicks

*2 Sickling in the skin*
Blood vessel blocked with sickled blood.

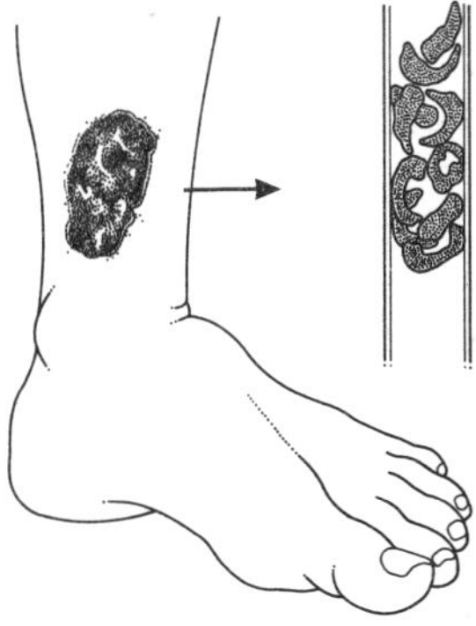

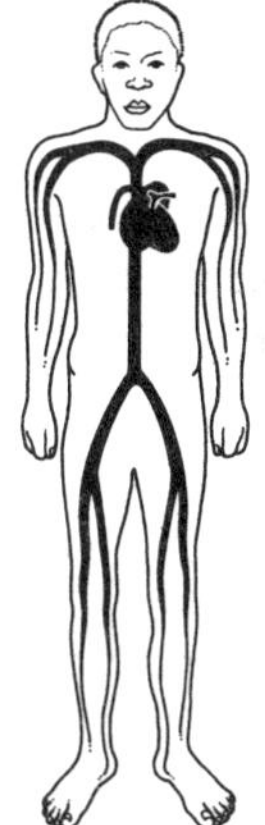

*3 Pressure on veins*
120–150 cm column of blood rests on the veins at the ankle.

Lying down – blood returns easily to the heart and the pressure is released from the veins at the ankle.

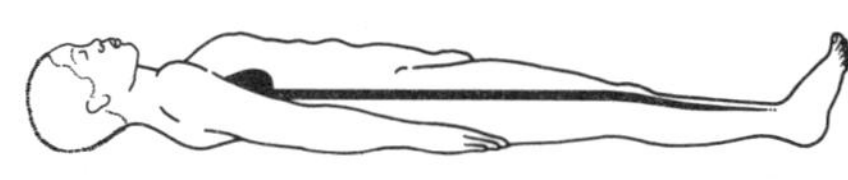

**Fig. 3** Causes of leg ulcers in sickle cell disease

the venous side of the blood circulation (i.e. the side returning blood to the heart and lungs) of the ankle is higher because of the effects of gravity and this will mean that blood flow through the skin of the ankle will be less good than say the skin of the forearm. The ankle is also a part of the body that is very easily knocked when walking about causing minor degrees of injury. It is also an area where ulcers due to varicose veins commonly occur so that it is a very sensitive area where healing of skin is particularly difficult. Sickle cell leg ulcers do not usually have an obvious preceding injury but may do so. What usually happens is that an area of skin becomes irritable and tender and sore. It is very important at this point that the area is protected and not scratched although this is obviously difficult to avoid. The skin over the ankle is then likely to become very dry and tough and then may split. This is usually the beginning of an ulcer and the split then opens up and spreads so that a sore develops. This can be quite deep going right through the skin showing fat in the base. The size is very variable and can be quite large although the usual size is about 2–3 $cm^2$.

Leg ulcers are a major problem particularly in developing countries where they are the cause of a very great deal of lost schooling and hence employment prospects. In Jamaica leg ulcers affect up to 75 per cent of sickle cell disease sufferers at some time in their life but in the UK it is substantially less than this, being more like 10 per cent.

Small ulcers (less than 2 cm across) may respond to cleanliness, regular dressing and antibiotics. There are only a few things which have been shown to improve the healing of larger leg ulcers. These are bed rest and blood transfusions. Bed rest is remarkably effective at healing the ulcers but does have to be very rigorously enforced. On occasions with severe ulcers it may be necessary to admit patients to hospital for some weeks to get the healing going. Most of this effect is probably because of the improved blood flow through the ankle caused by it being elevated to the same level as the heart. This takes the pressure off the veins and blood flow is improved. However, there is also some evidence that bed rest can modify the sickling process and reduce the number of irreversibly sickled cells in the circulation.

The use of special dressings has often been advocated but it is the bed rest that is the most important aspect. Clearly it is very important to keep the wound free of infection and cleaned of any debris. The use of skin grafts can be very effective in speeding up the healing, but this is usually only really useful when combined with exchange blood transfusion and bed rest.

Occasionally because of domestic circumstances or sometimes because of the severity of the ulcer it is necessary to resort to exchange blood transfusions to aid healing of the ulcer. This can be useful if an individual is at risk of losing a job and it will be very difficult for them to find another. It is usually possible to manage only smaller ulcers in this way but it can be very effective. Certainly a combination of exchange transfusions and bed rest leads to rapid resolution of the great majority of ulcers without the need to resort to skin grafting.

Prevention of leg ulcers is rather difficult but certainly sickle cell patients should be advised that they should endeavour to protect their ankles. This can be by using ankle length boots or protective splints. These are not usually cosmetically very acceptable therefore compliance is usually poor in those individuals who have not had problems with ulcers. Another useful way to try to prevent injury to the ankles is to advise the wearing of flat-soled shoes so that there is no sharp heel to catch the ankle while walking or running. In addition when the skin is hard and dry over the area and an ulcer is threatening to develop the use of skin softening creams and oils may have some value. Once the skin has broken down and the ulcer has developed this is not usually effective in the healing process.

## PROBLEMS RELATED TO SICKLING

### The Kidneys

The function of the kidney is to filter the blood and remove waste products so that these may be excreted in the urine. Urine is concentrated in the kidneys so that a relatively small amount of urine is passed for the amount of waste products removed. In order to fulfil its functions the kidney has a very good blood supply and is usually a well oxygenated organ. However, in order to develop the concentration of the urine there are areas of the kidney in which the salt concentration (osmolality) is very high and even in the presence of a quite high oxygen level if there is a very high salt concentration then the haemoglobin in the red cells may sickle causing damage to this part of the kidney. So potent is this effect of high salt concentration that even red cells from people with sickle cell trait will sickle under these circumstances and cause kidney problems. The problems specifically regarding sickle cell trait have been discussed in Chapter 2. Damage to the filtering mechanism of the kidney (glomeruli) also occurs in sickle cell disease but much later in life and is a more chronic process. A proportion of individuals with sickle cell disease will develop failure of the kidneys in late adolescence and early adulthood with an increasing incidence throughout life. At the present time there have been insufficient studies for a precise figure of the risk of kidney failure in adults with sickle cell disease to be produced.

## Kidney Function in Sickle Cell Disease

The usual ways in which kidney function is determined in man is to measure the levels of two substances, urea and creatinine, in the blood. These substances are filtered out of the blood by the kidneys and excreted in the urine. In sickle cell disease the levels of urea and creatinine in the blood are reduced, in particular the urea which is usually much below the normal range for healthy adults. Individuals with sickle cell disease have a high rate of filtering through the kidneys (a high glomerular filtration rate). This means that large amounts of urea are excreted. One of the earliest signs of kidney failure is an increase in the urea and creatinine in the blood but in sickle cell disease the increase in the urea and creatinine may be very small and well within the normal range for normal healthy adults. For this reason it is important to monitor the kidney function of sickle cell patients so that any small increase in urea can be detected early and management and diagnosis of any possible kidney problems commenced.

The other aspect of kidney function in sickle cell disease is the large volume of urine produced. This is because of the damage to the tubules that are responsible for concentrating the urine. In humans there is usually a variation in urine output over 24 hours so that at night less urine is produced. This works via a hormone called antidiuretic hormone which works on the distal kidney tubules. Since these tubules have been irreparably damaged in sickle cell disease this hormone has no target on which to work and therefore there is no reduction in urine output at night. This can lead to problems with bed wetting. This occurs both in sickle cell trait and in sickle cell disease. There is no treatment for the high urine output and any bed wetting problems are usually grown out of in later adoscelence. The problem with the large volumes of urine produced and the lack of sensitivity of the kidney to antidiuretic hormone means that when a patient with sickle cell disease becomes unwell and cannot drink enough fluid the kidney is unable to respond to the antidiuretic hormone by shutting down urine production. Urine continues to be produced in large amounts and the patient becomes more and more dehydrated and the sickling gets worse as the blood becomes more concentrated. In this way patients with sickle cell disease can easily become depleted of between 4 and 6 litres of fluid in quite a short period of time during a painful crisis or infection. Alcohol may promote the production of urine making dehydration more likely and excess alcohol usage is a predisposing factor in sickle cell painful crisis. Patients with sickle cell disease should be cautious in their use of alcohol and avoid becoming inebriated.

*Haematuria* (Blood in the Urine)

Most of the time the damage to the tubules in the kidneys takes place in a very slow and chronic way with tiny amounts of damage occurring at any one time. The changes are completely unknown to the patient. However, on occasions the sickling is more severe in this area and pieces of kidney actually die and become necrotic. These may fall off of the papillae of the kidney into the urine causing bleeding as they do so. Therefore pain in the loins and bleeding into the urine is not uncommon in sickle cell disease. However, in any individual with sickle cell disease or sickle trait who has blood in their urine it is important for medical staff to exclude any more serious cause such as an infection or bladder warts which may be treatable in the early stages. In the UK, haematuria (blood in the urine) appears to be quite unusual in sickle cell disease sufferers but certainly the damage to the kidney tubules is not and the inability to concentrate the urine is a universal finding.

## Chronic Renal Failure

Damage to the kidney tubules does not normally lead to significant kidney failure. However, if the damage is extended into the areas where the glomeruli occur then the ability of the kidney to filter urea and creatinine and other by-products of the body is reduced and chronic renal failure may develop. Very significant losses of kidney function can occur with minimal increases in urea and creatinine. Because these chemicals are already low in the blood of sickle cell disease sufferers, by the time it is noticed that the urea and creatinine are increasing very major kidney damage has occurred. Why some individuals get kidney failure and others do not is unknown. It has been noted that many patients who do get kidney failure are less severely affected sickle cell patients who have a high rate of haemolysis in the blood. There may be some toxic by-product of haemolysis occurring. But this appears to be less likely than sickling within the glomerular areas causing specific local damage.

Once kidney failure develops it tends to progress quite quickly and patients often require kidney dialysis within a year or two of initial diagnosis. The management of the kidney failure needs to be dealt with in its own right by a skilled renal physician working in collaboration with the haematologist. Kidney transplantation is certainly an option for these patients but of course the sickle cell disease is still present and will lead to some damage to the transplanted kidney even if there is no rejection.

## Bone and Joint Disease

Painful crises occur regularly in the bones. At the time of the episode it is usually not possible to see any changes on the radiograph. As the years go by the damage to the bones becomes very evident with characteristic changes of increased bone formation and density detectable by X-ray. Recent investigation using magnetic resonance imaging has shown infarcted areas of bone (i.e. areas which are starved of blood) very soon after a sickle cell crisis. However, this technique is not widely available and is unlikely to be helpful in the diagnosis and management of painful crises. In adults most bone infarcts occur away from joints and do not cause any major problems but this is not the case in children. While the bone is growing it is possible for a sickle crisis to occur near to or at the growing point of the bone causing permanent damage. Such damage means that the bone will cease to grow. Happily this occurs only very rarely with long limb bones but is most commonly seen in bones of the hands and feet. This can lead to the sickle cell patient having a short finger or toe. In children damage to the bones of the hands and feet lead to painful swelling and the so-called hand–foot syndrome. This will be discussed in more detail in Chapter 8.

In both children and adults increased bone growth occurs because of the expanding marrow cavity within the bone. This can be particularly prominent when it affects the bones of the skull, producing a very prominent forehead appearance which is quite characteristic of chronic haemolytic anaemia. The very long-term problem with bones in sickle cell disease is damage to the major weight-bearing joints. This particularly affects the hip joints but also the shoulders. Damage to the hip joint can be either chronic (i.e. continuous) damage or due to an acute infarct. In an acute case a previously well, usually young, adult with sickle cell disease is admitted with a severe crisis involving pain in one or both hips. As the crisis resolves the pain in the hip is not relieved and movement is reduced. After a week or so radiographic changes in the hip become apparent and it is obvious that the bone of the head and neck of the femur is dead. This leads to pain and instability in the hip and limitation of movement. Sometimes mobilization can be achieved but often this is not possible particularly if the hip is unstable. It is then necessary to proceed directly to total hip replacement. An alternative is to fix in the hip in one position but this does not preserve any useful function in the hip. The immediate postoperative benefits of total hip replacement are usually excellent. The main reservation about total hip replacement in sickle cell disease relates to the long-term outlook. Technically the hip replacement operation is difficult since the chronic damage to the bone of the pelvis and the rest of the hip makes it quite difficult to chisel and mould the bone to accept the hip replacement. Most patients, however, have quite a good result in the intermediate term but the long-term results will have to await many more years of follow-up before they can be properly assessed.

Similar problems can occur with the knees and shoulders with chronic sickling occurring at these points leading to a breakdown in the surfaces of the bone and pain and limitation of movement. Shoulders and knees cannot readily be replaced and treatment has focused on managing the sickle cell patient as a whole to try and enable them to come to terms with their disability and to adapt their lifestyle accordingly. Bone joint surgery in sickle cell disease is a major undertaking because of the difficulty of working the bone because of its hardness. Because of this it is essential that the patient should be adequately prepared with transfusion therapy.

## Strokes

Sickling in the brain is quite a rare occurrence although it can occur in association with a very severe generalized sickling crisis. It is sometimes associated with chest or girdle syndrome.

One manifestation of sickling in the brain is a stroke. Stroke results when sickling in a blood vessel causes it to be blocked and the section of brain supplied by that blood vessel dies. This produces either weakness or a speech defect, depending upon which part of the body that section of the brain deals with. It is quite common for normal individuals to have slight differences in the blood vessel pattern in their brain and it is thought that those individuals who have strokes in association with sickle cell disease may have a slightly abnormal blood vessel pattern in their brain. These are called arteriovenous malformations and do seem to predispose sickle cell sufferers to strokes. One of the problems with strokes in sickle cell disease is that they do tend to recur particularly in children. For this reason it is felt appropriate to institute a regime of exchange transfusion for any sickle cell patient who has a stroke in childhood. At the present time the transfusions tend to be given at six-weekly intervals for about two years but there is a case to be made out for continuing for longer. There is a fear that the risk of stroke is only delayed and not prevented by transfusions.

## Liver Disease in Sickle Cell Disease

Most of the problems related to the liver in sickle cell disease have been considered in the discussion of haemolytic anaemia. Jaundice is a common finding in sickle cell disease patients. This does not usually signify problems with liver malfunction, but is a consequence of the increased destruction of red blood cells leading to increased production of bilirubin.

Gall-stones occur with much increased frequency because of the increased turnover of bilirubin. Occasionally symptoms similar to those produced by gall-stones occur but no gall-stones can be identified on ultrasound scan. In these cases it is often the bile itself that has become so thick that the duct becomes blocked and the liver increases in size and becomes tender. The patient becomes severely jaundiced. This problem is sometimes seen in pregnant women with sickle cell disease.

The spleen filters bacteria and old red cells from the blood. In sickle cell disease patients the function of the spleen is usually lost by the age of five years. The liver then takes on many of the functions of the spleen, in particular the breakdown and removal of red blood cells from the circulation. Biopsies of livers from patients with sickle cell disease therefore often show increased numbers of sickle cell within the liver, which is often enlarged because of the increased numbers of red blood cells within it. Occasionally these red cell numbers may become greatly increased in a manner similar to splenic sequestration. In this case the liver becomes rapidly enlarged and fills with blood and the treatment will be exactly the same as for sequestration involving the spleen (see p. 24).

Patients who receive prolonged transfusions of blood will be prone to suffer from iron overload if they are not treated adequately with the drug desferrioxamine. Iron overload may cause iron toxicity in the liver including cirrhosis. Other problems related to such long-term blood transfusion therapy include virus hepatitis which can also be a factor in the development of cirrhosis of the liver.

## Problems Related to Splenic Atrophy

### *Infections*

In childhood the spleen acts as an important organ and plays a part in developing antibodies to certain bacteria and foreign agents. In normal individuals the importance of the function of the spleen seems to decrease through life and it is certainly possible to remove the spleen after the age of five years without any major consequences to the overall development of the immune system.

The spleen is a smallish organ about 18 × 13 × 7 cm (7 × 5 × 3 in) and consists mainly of blood and lymph gland tissues. In many ways it resembles a tonsil but with more blood in it. Blood flow through the spleen is slow and the oxygen tension is low. Therefore, for individuals with sickle cell disease there is ample opportunity for cell sickling to occur within the spleen. It is believed that this does indeed occur and that progressive splenic damage takes place from the time in the first year of life when sickle cell haemoglobin becomes the major component of the blood. As the spleen becomes more and more damaged its function deteriorates so that by the age of five years most splenic function has been lost.

The function of the spleen that is lost is the filtering out of small particles. The spleen is an important area for removing blood cells that have become old or damaged. Blood has to squeeze through very narrow pores within the spleen and there are also receptors on the cells which can react with foreign bodies. The most serious consequence of the loss of splenic function is the inability to filter out certain bacteria, particularly pneumococcus, meningococcus and salmonella. These abnormalities are not peculiar to individuals with sickle cell disease but occur in anyone who has had their spleen removed. This means that they are at constant risk of overwhelming infection from meningococcus and pneumococcus and also have an increased risk of certain infections, particularly osteomyelitis, caused by salmonella organisms. The risk of pneumococcal and meningococcal infections is so great that it is recommended that children take penicillin 250 mg twice a day until adulthood. The risk of developing these infections is great where large bodies of people are present together, for instance schools, universities and the armed forces. The idea behind taking the penicillin until, say, twenty-one years of age is that by then most individuals will have left those environments where they are most likely to acquire such infections. However, there is a small but significant risk of further meningococcal or pneumococcal infections throughout life and a good case can be made that individuals who have had their spleen removed or have lost spleen function because of sickle cell disease should continue to take pencillin for life.

Recent concerns in Britain regarding salmonella in eggs should be taken seriously by sickle cell patients, especially children. Eggs should be well cooked to ensure there is no risk of exposure to salmonella.

Although individuals with sickle cell trait have some resistance to malaria, particularly falciparum malaria, this is not the case in individuals with sickle cell disease. One of the body's other natural defences against malaria is that the malaria parasites are filtered out in the spleen. In the absence of any functioning spleen malarial infections can rapidly become overwhelming and it is therefore imperative that individuals with sickle disease take antimalarial medication whenever in a malarial zone.

FIVE

# Pain Relief

Pain is a regular companion to most patients with sickle cell disease. Many of them come to fear the pain and to dread the inadequate analgesia that so many of them endure in hospital. The management of pain by medical staff and patients themselves is essential to the successful care of sickle cell disease patients.

Pain relief in sickle cell disease must be considered in relation to the patient's location (i.e. home or hospital) and why the pain is present. It is also important to consider the likely duration of the pain. The approach will differ if it is related to an acute sickle cell crisis or due to chronic damage to a joint, or to leg ulcers.

Painful sickle cell crises are the commonest cause of short periods of severe pain in sickle cell disease. Episodes of gall-stone colic can also give rise to short periods of severe pain. Individuals with sickle cell disease are, of course, just as likely as any other person to develop appendicitis or other acute abdominal problems. These must be ruled out by doctors before powerful painkillers are given because the effect of drugs like pethidine is to mask the signs of these conditions and can lead to them being overlooked until serious complications have set in and the patient is seriously ill.

Chronic pain is most commonly due to joint damage related to previous bone infarcts particularly in the hip joint. Other forms of chronic pain are due to gall bladder pain from gall-stones and inflammation of the gall bladder, and to sickle cell leg ulcers.

## Analgesia Dependence

The exposure of sickle cell sufferers to pain on a regular basis means that they come into contact with pain-killers – analgesics –

frequently. The painkillers are often powerful opiate drugs. There is therefore a potential problem of dependence on painkilling drugs. In fact this appears to be remarkably uncommon in the UK and the great majority of individuals have no difficulty withdrawing from even very large doses of potent opiate analgesics following recovery from painful sickle cell crises. A small proportion of severely affected individuals may have difficulty weaning off these high doses and may need support from a Drug Dependency Unit or Sickle Cell Counselling Services.

## PAIN MANAGEMENT IN SICKLE CELL CRISIS

Patients may develop a sickle cell crisis pain that can be managed at home or requires hospital admission.

### Management at Home

Patients can learn how to manage minor sickle cell crises at home. Many patients do so in any event after becoming disenchanted with frequent visits and admissions to hospital. They can get help to manage their sickle cell crisis at home with advice from the hospital or Sickle Cell Counselling Service. This ensures that a standardized management system is instituted. When patients do present at hospital it is then immediately apparent to doctors how they have been treating themselves up to that time.

Because of the risks of drug misuse and habituation, the exact regime of analgesics to be used at home needs to be considered with some care. The sublingual (sprayed under the tongue) agent Temgesic (buprenorphine) is useful because it is quite a potent analgesic, but induces significant feelings of nausea and sickness. This makes habituation unlikely. There is no euphoriant effect but the analgesia is quite potent and effective. The nausea can be combated with agents such as prochlorperazine (Stematil) or metoclopromide (Maxolon). Another agent commonly used at home is dihydrocodeine (DF118) but this does have a significant risk of habituation and dependency when used frequently. Any patients managing their own sickle cell crisis at home must maintain a very high fluid intake and keep themselves warm and dry. They should be confident in the knowledge that they have immediate access to hospital attention where they can be quickly assessed and where admission can be arranged if necessary. Alternatively they can contact their general practitioner for additional advice. The general practitioner may decide to use a few doses of a more potent injectable analgesic such as pethidine or morphine at home before considering referral to hospital. Any sickle cell crisis that is not improving within 48 hours or has high fever (over 38.5°C) or breathing difficulty must be referred to hospital either by the patients themselves or their general practitioner.

## Management of Sickle Cell Crises in Hospital

The cornerstone of management in hospital is the rapid attention to the patient on arrival and the rapid administration of analgesia. However, good medical practice requires that a diagnosis is made so that any surgical or acute medical causes not related to sickle cell disease are excluded before powerful analgesic drugs are given. Otherwise these painkillers might mask any symptoms and signs of other disorders. Full explanation to the patient of what is happening is also important, and the patient should feel free to ask for an explanation of the treatment used. This engenders a feeling of confidence and support so that the patient can feel that his or her pain is going to be relieved shortly. Ideally patients should be nursed on a ward which is familiar with sickle cell disease and used to administering the pain-relieving regimes. It is useful if a relationship has been built up between nursing staff, medical staff and patients over the years.

## Analgesia Regimes

The standard regimen for inpatient analgesia in the UK has been intramuscular injections of pethidine of 100 mg up to 1½–2 hourly intervals. Injections must be clearly written up by the doctor as '2 hourly' and not 'as required'. This is an effective regime in the majority of moderate sickle cell crises but it is often inadequate in severe crises. It also has a number of problems. First, pethidine is a very short-acting analgesic; although it does work very promptly it also wears off quickly. It also has a very strong euphoriant effect and individuals can come to look forward to this boost making habituation and weaning off more difficult than with some other agents. Furthermore, pethidine has irritant effects on the nervous system and can cause epileptic fits when levels in the blood become high. A study at the Central Middlesex Hospital showed that regular injection of pethidine frequently leads to levels in the blood which are potentially harmful, with the risk of fits.

An alternative method of administering pethidine is by an infusion pump. This can be effective and the euphoriant effect is less marked. However, many patients find that infusion pumps are less satisfactory than giving intermittent intramuscular analgesics. The latter are very demanding for nursing staff to give, particularly if many patients are admitted at the same time. Morphine infusion pumps can be used but in our experience in Birmingham these have not been very successful. This may relate to the slower onset of analgesia and attention to the initial control of analgesia is most important. Probably the optimum method of management is to induce analgesia quickly and effectively with intravenous or intramuscular injections of morphine or pethidine and to follow this up with an infusion pump which also allows the patient to administer additional booster doses on demand (patient-controlled analgesia systems). The frequency of the booster doses can be controlled by the medical attendants so that the total dose of opiates given is not excessive.

## Reducing Analgesics

This must be done in full consultation between patients, medical and nursing staff. It can be difficult to establish a specific regime for reducing the analgesic dose as the patient recovers by, for example, halving the amount of pethidine on a daily or every other daily basis. However, it is often possible to substitute directly from injectable opiates to drugs taken by mouth, in particular long-acting morphine derivatives or dihydrocodeine. This works best if the pain resolution is particularly rapid. Most patients will be able to leave hospital on no analgesics or at most dihydrocodeine. It should be very rarely necessary for patients to be discharged with a small supply of pethidine. It should not be necesary for a patient to be discharged with more than ten doses of pethidine.

## Improving the Pain Relief

There are other techniques that can be used in combination with the opiate analgesics to increase the overall pain relief.

### *Other Drugs*

These include non-steroidal anti-inflammatory agents (NSAIDs) such as indomethacin and ibuprofen. These are sometimes dramatically helpful for patients with bone pain but in many patients are completely ineffective. **Chlorpromazine** reinforces and potentiates the effect of opiate analgesics. Care must be taken in its use with pethidine since together the risk of epileptic fits is increased. Patients should be fully informed as to why and when they are to start chlorpromazine because of its sedative effects. Patients with sickle cell disease do not in the main like feeling 'drugged up' and chlorpromazine is one agent that does produce this effect very strongly. Another agent that is sometimes useful is **diazepam (Valium)** which can be useful soon after admission to hospital for patients who are also highly anxious as well as in pain. However, it is not usually helpful in the longer term since it does not have an analgesic effect, but only removes the memory of the pain (amnesic effect). It also produces a suppressing effect on the brain.

### *TENS*

Another way in which pain may be alleviated, particularly if it is associated with a single joint or bony area, is the use of a transcutaneous nerve stimulator (TENS). This works by passing a weak electric current across the painful area. This can be dramatically helpful in some patients and appears to act by a counter irritation principle, i.e. the current causes an irritation that cancels out the pain. The method is harmless and non-addictive but unfortunately each machine costs approximately £100 and the cost is a barrier to providing machines for home use.

*Heat*

In hospital, the use of electric heat pads is much appreciated by patients. The heat pad is placed on the back or over the knees or whichever is the most painful part. Of course, patients should also be nursed in a warm dry environment to minimize the risk of further sickling.

## Chronic Pain Relief

The main causes of chronic pain in sickle cell disease have been discussed in Chapters 3 and 4. Obviously, the control of pain should concentrate on the treatment and attempted cure of the underlying problem. For instance if pain is very severe from a hip joint, total hip replacement will be considered. If the pain is from leg ulcers then active aggressive management of the leg ulcers to assist healing should be instituted immediately by medical staff. Sometimes there may be reasons why surgery or treatment of a particular complication is not appropriate and management of chronic pain at home is required. In these instances the first treatment should be with NSAIDs (see p.44) such as ibuprofen, in order to avoid the risk of opiate dependence. Other drugs of intermediate strength such as dihydrocodeine are often helpful in orthopaedic situations, especially in combination with aspirin or other NSAIDs. Potent opiates such as long-acting morphine or pethidine should be reserved for very severe pain not responding to any other measures.

## Attitudes to Analgesia

Attitudes towards providing analgesia for sickle cell disease is an area of serious conflict between medical staff, including nurses and sickle cell patients. A recent study showed that sickle cell sufferers consider that the severity of the pain endured in a sickle cell crisis is consistently underestimated by the carers. The sufferers scored their pain at about 8 out of 10 on a scale of 10 whereas they felt that the carers viewed the pain at the 2 or 3 level. Clearly, sickle cell patients think that the doctors and nurses do not take their pain sufficiently seriously. The main concern of sickle cell sufferers is that the pain is not relieved quickly, nor comprehensively enough. One of the advantages of a patient-controlled analgesia system is that the patients know best the pain they are experiencing although the dosages obviously must be kept within safe margins by medical attendants. It is extremely important that analgesia is given promptly as soon as alternative causes of the pain have been excluded. Patients should have open access to present themselves immediately to a ward where doctors and nurses with expertise in the subject are readily available to attend to them. This does not necessarily exclude the general practitioner from managing the patient but recognizes the fact that sickle cell disease patients know their

**Table 2** Control of pain

| | |
|---|---|
| 1 *Painful sickle cell crisis* | |
| Mild – moderate | Paracetamol, Co-proxamol<br>Buprenorphine (Temgesic)<br>Dihydrocodeine<br>Pethidine or morphine tablets |
| Severe | Pethidine or morphine<br>intramuscular injections<br>intravenous infusion pump (ideally with patient-controlled analgesia)<br>subcutaneous infusions<br>use together with<br>chlorpromazine or diazepam<br>NSAID<br>Heat and/or TENS |
| 2 *Chronic pain* | |
| Treat the underlying cause | |
| Use drugs that will not produce dependence whenever possible | |
| | Paracetamol<br>NSAIDs |

condition and can tell quickly when they will be unable to manage at home. There is no good reason why a patient with sickle cell disease should not expect to have their pain relieved within 30 minutes of arriving at hospital. Their pain should thereafter remain relieved or at a tolerable level for the remainder of their inpatient stay however long this should be. Instances of drug dependence occurring after an acute crisis are virtually unknown and there is no good reason for medical and nursing staff to disbelieve individuals with sickle cell disease as regards the severity of their plan. It is most important to devise a pain relief regime that works efficiently and to ensure that these facilities are made available to the patient as soon and as reliably as possible.

SIX

# Blood Transfusion

## GENERAL PRINCIPLES

Patients with sickle cell disease usually have a low haemoglobin level (anaemia), but this in itself is not a reason for blood transfusion. As explained in Chapter 1, for a given haemoglobin level an increased amount of oxygen is delivered to the body tissues by sickle haemoglobin. It is therefore unusual for patients to suffer from a lack of oxygen during the steady state. Blood transfusions should only be considered in specific instances. Furthermore, because there are numerous complications related to blood transfusion (including overloading the body with iron, development of antibodies to red cells and the transmission of viral infections) they should only be considered to deal with specific conditions.

There is an additional problem with blood transfusions that is specific to sickle cell disease. The blood cells in sickle cell are stiffer than usual. This means that the thickness or viscosity of blood in sickle cell disease is approximately the same as that of normal blood, even though the haemoglobin may only be half the level of that in a normal person. If transfusions of normal blood are given on top of the sickle haemoglobin this will lead to a substantial increase in the whole blood viscosity and potentially worsen the sickling complication for which the transfusion is being given. On occasions it is safe and appropriate simply to top up with a blood transfusion, such as in an anaemic crisis or sequestration crisis but these will usually be associated with a very low haemoglobin of less than about 4 g/dl (normal haemoglobin level is 6 to 9 g/dl). During blood transfusion regimes in sickle cell disease it is important for doctors to monitor the percentage of haemoglobin S in the blood and also the haematocrit (proportion of red blood cells by volume in the blood). Previous studies have shown that if the percentage of sickle haemoglobin and the haematocrit are too high then this can lead to a sickle cell crisis. If the percentage haemoglobin S in the blood is multiplied by the haematocrit a figure called the sicklecrit is obtained. Provided this is kept below 15 per cent it is safe to transfuse without removing any blood. If the figure for the sicklecrit is greater than 15 per cent, however, exchange transfusion should be carried out (see p. 55).

Haematocrit × % Hb S = Sicklecrit (%)

## COMPLICATIONS OF BLOOD TRANSFUSION

### Iron overload

One pint (or unit) of blood contains approximately 250 mg of iron. Regular blood transfusions will lead to an increase of iron in the body, because there is no normal system for the removal of iron from the body. In patients who need regular blood transfusions over two years or more, iron loading in the body can be quite substantial. It is then deposited in vital organs such as the heart, liver, pancreas and other endocrine glands. In time this can lead to problems with heart failure, liver disease and diabetes. Children may not go through puberty because of damage to the ovaries or testes. In addition, individuals with haemolytic anaemias such as sickle cell disease tend to absorb iron more efficiently from the blood than from their food and therefore have an intrinsic tendency to accumulate iron. All patients with sickle cell disease should have their iron status monitored every year or so to ensure that they are not getting increased levels of iron in the body. This can be done quite readily by measuring levels of serum ferritin, a substance in the blood which accurately reflect stores of iron in the body. Patients having transfusions should have their ferritin levels measured more frequently.

If patients are having numerous transfusions and have had more than 30 or 40 units of blood transfused in their life, they will be considered for treatment to remove iron from the body. This is quite difficult and at the present time can only be done reliably with infusions of a drug called desferrioxamine. The desferrioxamine is injected slowly just under the skin (subcutaneously) using a small pump over a ten to twelve hour period. This must be done on at least five nights a week (ideally seven) so that the patient's life is not disrupted unduly. However, it is still a very restricting treatment and moderately uncomfortable.

Because of these problems with iron overload, large volume blood transfusion regimes should only be undertaken for very good reasons and following full discussion between the patient and medical staff. Usually individuals requiring desferrioxamine will have serum ferritin levels greater than 3000 mg/litre and therapy should be continued until the ferritin has come down below 2000 mg/litre and the requirement for blood transfusions has ceased. If blood transfusion is proposed on a longterm basis desferrioxamine therapy should continue throughout this period. There are some exciting developments in drugs that remove iron, and can be taken by mouth (oral chelators) though at the present time these remain experimental. They may not be able to reduce iron loading in patients who are overloaded already, but could have a major impact in the early stages of iron overload by preventing its occurrence.

## Red Cell Antibodies

Because most individuals with sickle cell disease are of Afro-Caribbean origin they tend to inherit a number of minor blood group systems which are slightly different from those in other parts of the world. For example in technical terms they rarely express antigens of the CE rhesus group system and are nearly always Lewis and Duffy blood groups negative. This means that such individuals, when in a community consisting of a majority of Caucasians, will tend to receive blood products that have been donated by white people who have a high incidence of rhesus CE, Lewis and Duffy antigens. Transfusion with such blood is likely to lead to the production of antibodies to these groups by the sickle cell patient.

Another important blood group is Kell. Almost all black people are negative for Kell and the majority of white people are positive. This means that blood must be very carefully screened and cross matched before being administered to individuals with sickle cell disease. In order to prevent some of these problems, it has been proposed that sickle cell sufferers should receive only blood that is Rhesus CE and Kell negative, but this has not been accepted generally in the UK.

## Virus Transmission

In the UK and most other developed countries all blood products are screened for hepatitis B and the human immunodeficiency virus (HIV). However, screening is not available for non A, non B(NANB) hepatitis which is commonly transmitted by blood products. (One type of NANB hepatitis is now called hepatitis C.) Although relatively rare in the UK, NANB hepatitis can cause jaundice and hepatitis and on rare occasions can cause chronic liver disease. Although it is extremely unlikely that hepatitis B or HIV will be transmitted by blood transfusions in the UK, it does remain a remote possibility. Blood transfusions should therefore only be administered after careful consideration of the possible consequences and the reasons for the transfusion. In many other parts of the world, for reasons of cost, it is not possible to test blood transfusions for viral transmission. If testing is not adequate where the blood has been collected then the risk of virus transmission must be considered seriously. The reasons for blood transfusion would be substantially reduced and would be limited to life-saving situations only.

## Venous Access

Patients with sickle cell disease often require repeated admissions to hospital during which they may require intravenous drips to administer fluids. These episodes occur particularly in childhood and damage to veins may occur. By the time patients reach late adolescence or early adult life it may be difficult to find veins to take blood and to administer intravenous fluids. Approximately 10 per cent of individuals with sickle cell disease have significant problems with access to their veins. In the great majority of cases it is possible to continue treatment using veins in the arms without resorting to other veins in the legs. Also modern techniques enable safe and confident access to large veins in the upper chest by placing plastic tubes (catheters) into them through the skin. Some patients may have severe and persistent problems with poor veins. This can be a threat to their life by preventing adequate management of severe problems. For these patients it is possible to insert semi-permanent indwelling devices that can be accessed by medical staff. These devices should not be inserted without much thought, since they act as a potential source of infection. Rigorous sterile technique is essential whenever using the device. The most commonly used indwelling device is a Port-a-Cath which can be accessed through the skin and which leaves no part of the device outside the body. It can safely be left in place for five years or more.

## REASONS FOR BLOOD TRANSFUSIONS

Blood transfusions are required for the short term to cover urgent operations (an acute cause), to support a patient through a pregnancy or to allow leg ulcers to heal (elective or subacute transfusion regime). Certain conditions require long-term therapy, for example, an episode of stroke (cerebrovascular sickling), severe persisting sickle cell crises or kidney failure.

### Short-term Transfusions

*Acute Transfusion Requirements*

1 Chest syndrome
2 Severe persistent crisis. Crisis lasting more than 7 days with no evidence of improvement.
3 Surgical emergency
4 Anaemic crisis (diagnosed by fall in reticulocytes and a haemoglobin usually <4 g/dl)
5 Sequestration crisis

The items 1, 2 and 3 must be managed by exchange transfusion whereas anaemic crisis and sequestration crisis can be managed by simple top up transfusion. It is particularly important in sequestration crisis that concentrated (packed) red cells are used for the transfusion prior to any salt solutions being infused. Once the decision to transfuse has been taken it is important to monitor the percentage of haemoglobin S and to maintain the sicklecrit at less than 15 per cent. In an emergency it may be necessary for a patient to undergo surgery before blood can be made available and an exchange transfusion started. In such a situation the following plan should be followed:

1 *Rehydrate the patient before surgery.* It is particularly important that the patient receives intravenous fluids during the period that they are fasting before the operation.
2 *Oxygen.* During the operation the patient must be kept well oxygenated and following the operation, oxygen (40 per cent) must continue to be administered and this must be supervised by an identified person. This is to prevent the sleepy patient knocking the oxygen mask from their face.
3 *Physiotherapy.* Chest physiotherapy should be instituted soon after returning the patient to the ward and early mobilization is most important to encourage good oxygenation and blood supply to the lungs.
4 *Prevention of Thrombosis.* Patients who might be expected to have a long period of rest in bed or who are on the contraceptive pill should receive subcutaneous heparin to prevent deep vein thrombosis.

*Elective Transfusion*

Elective transfusion means that some planning can be involved in the timing of non-urgent surgery such as gall bladder removal. This also applies to the therapy for leg ulcers and for pregnancy. A study for King's College Hospital has shown that individuals undergoing surgery for gall bladder removal do much better and have less infections and pneumonia if they are transfused beforehand so that the sickle haemoglobin is less than 30 per cent.

Pregnancy has been a controversial area for blood transfusions in sickle cell disease. There are two schools of thought, one believing that transfusions are important in managing pregnancy and the other that it has no place. A recent trial from the United States showed no benefit from transfusions in pregnancy but this may not always be the case. Late in pregnancy it is quite common for the haemoglobin level to fall and it is then necessary to transfuse the patient urgently. Transfusions are still important for the pregnant woman with severe sickle cell disease, particularly when sickle crises have already occurred or previous severe problems have been encountered. If a transfusion regime is to be used in a pregnancy the best time to start has to be decided. This will be either as soon as possible after conception or from approximately 28 weeks. Most problems occur after 28 weeks but the development of the placenta and infant will get most benefit by transfusion from soon after conception. A compromise is to begin transfusions after the first sickling complication. It is usually adequate to transfuse the patients over several weeks. Initially two exchanges in the first four to five days can be followed by weekly exchanges for the next three to four weeks until the percentage of sickle cell haemoglobin is less than 30 per cent. Top up transfusions can be administered after that.

Severe leg ulcers respond very well to blood transfusion. They also respond to bed rest, but it is often difficult for patients to rest for as long as is needed for the ulcers to heal. Transfusions do have the benefit for some individuals that schooling, education or work can continue while their leg ulcers are healing.

## Long-term Transfusion Regimes

The aim should be to keep the sickle haemoglobin percentage below 30 per cent at all times. Once the Hb S level is less than this a transfusion of three to four units of blood every four weeks should be sufficient to keep it there. Desferrioxamine treatment must be given at the same time to remove iron from the body. The following are examples of some conditions for which long-term blood transfusion may be necessary.

1 Stroke. Transfuse for at least two years following a stroke and if it has occurred in a child consider continuing until adolescence.
2 Severe recurrent crises. The patient can be given a break from recurrent crises by maintaining the sickle level below 20 per cent for at least six months.
3 Bone disease. Destruction of bones such as the hips may respond and settle with a 'wait and see' approach and a period of blood transfusion.
4 Education. This is very important as people with sickle cell disease are unlikely to be able to earn their living in physical work. Therefore a transfusion regime of one or two years may be appropriate to enable studies to be completed.
5 Leg ulcers. Patients who have recurrent leg ulcers that break down repeatedly may require longer-term transfusion.
6 Kidney failure. Kidney failure is a complication of sickle cell disease and is usually associated with a failure of production of red blood cells or erythropoietin by the kidney. This hormone stimulates the bone marrow to produce red blood cells and if the level of erythropoietin falls then worsening of the anaemia will result. If this occurs it may be essential to keep the haemoglobin at an adequate level with blood transfusions. Artificial erythropoietin is now available but the dose given in sickle cell disease has to be very precise to prevent the haemoglobin increasing too much and making the sickling problems worse.

## EXCHANGE BLOOD TRANSFUSION REGIME FOR NON-EMERGENCY OPERATION

An example of a transfusion regime for exchange transfusion of an urgent but non-emergency operation that needs to be done in the next week or so is given in Table 3. Before commencing the transfusions blood should be taken for serum ferritin to assess the body iron stores. It is also important to perform tests of liver function and to look for antibodies to hepatitis B and C and the human immunodeficiency virus (HIV). These tests must be discussed between doctor and patient beforehand, since they are carried out to confirm that there is no evidence of these viruses before the transfusions. If there is any concern in the future about any virus infection being acquired from a blood transfusion, these pre-transfusion tests will make the investigation of any infection much easier.

It is also possible to produce an excellent exchange transfusion using a cell separator machine exchanging between six and eight units of blood. In conditions such as chest syndrome it is sometimes difficult to carry out such an exchange on a cell separator because of inadequate blood flow and increased blood viscosity and in this situation it is essential to carry out a manual exchange. It may even be necessary to use a syringe to remove blood and inject it in.

**Table 3** Transfusion regime: urgent non-emergency exchange transfusion

| *Day* | *Blood removed* | *Blood given* | *Tests* |
|---|---|---|---|
| 1 | 2 units | 3–4 units | Haemoglobin<br>Haematocrit |
| 2 | 2 units | 4 units | Hb, %Hb S<br>Haematocrit<br>Sicklecrit |
| 3 | 2 units | 3 units | Hb, %Hb S<br>Haematocrit<br>Sicklecrit |
| 4 | 1 unit | 2 units | Hb, %Hb S<br>Haematocrit<br>Sicklecrit |
| 5 | nil | 1–3 units | Hb, %Hb S<br>Haematocrit<br>Sicklecrit |

SEVEN

# Sexual Problems in Sickle Cell Disease

For many years pregnancy for individuals with sickle cell disease was not considered possible and as recently as 1970 a conference suggested that for women with sickle cell disease the risks of pregnancy were so great as not to justify embarking on a pregnancy. However, over the last 15 years it has become apparent that women with sickle cell disease can complete successful pregnancies even though the rate of complications may be substantially increased over that of their healthy sisters. Issues of fertility, contraception and pregnancy have taken a major place in the management of sickle cell disease. In addition to these aspects there is one complication of sickle cell disease which affects the male, priapism, which requires specific discussion.

## FERTILITY

This was previously thought to be very low. However recent studies show that women with sickle cell disease do not have any significant difficulty in conceiving, although there is an increased risk of spontaneous abortion. There is some evidence that men are subfertile. This has a number of causes. First, there is a significant risk of impotence following episodes of serious priapism (see below). Second, there is a reduction in production of sperm (spermatogenesis) in men with sickle cell disease possibly related to testicular malfunction, the cause of which is not known. However, this certainly does not affect all males with sickle cell disease.

## PRIAPISM

The incidence of priapism among men with sickle cell disease is unknown but in patients in Birmingham is between 10 and 15 per cent. Priapism is defined as prolonged painful erection of the penis in the absence of sexual desire. Severe episodes may last for many hours and even into days in the most extreme cases. A history of preceding episodes of less severe priapism is quite common. These last for a few hours followed by spontaneous resolution and normal potency thereafter. It is important for patients to report previous episodes of priapism to medical staff as a routine since frequent recurring episodes can be treated to reduce erections. This may stave off a major episode of priapism.

An established case of severe priapism is an extremely painful disorder requiring potent analgesia. On occasions oral, intramuscular and intravenous analgesics are insufficient and spinal anaesthesia may be required. Medical management should be as for a painful sickle cell crisis with adequate rehydration and analgesics. There is no evidence to suggest that exchange transfusion is helpful and during the time taken to do this effectively it is likely that the erection would be lost.

Surgical intervention includes needling the penis under local anaesthetic and sucking out blood. This is often effective in the short term but recurrences within a few hours are quite common. Such a procedure can be repeated on a number of occasions during the same episode and if unsuccessful it may be necessary to proceed to a vein bypass procedure to decompress the penis. Individuals who have had episodes of major priapism or recurrent minor (stuttering) priapism may be considered by medical staff as needing management with an antitestosterone agent such as cyproterone acetate. The aim of this therapy is to reduce spontaneous erections in the hope that this will prevent another episode of priapism.

The outlook after priapism is variable but there is a significant risk of permanent impotence following major episodes lasting longer than 18–24 hours. Impotent individuals may need treatment with surgical prosthetic implants.

## CONTRACEPTION

Contraception is one of the most widely misunderstood areas in sickle cell disease. It is also one of the most important areas to get right, since although there are no absolute reasons why women with sickle cell disease should not become pregnant, complication rates are substantially increased and management can be quite complex. Therefore pregnancies in women with sickle cell disease are best planned in advance whenever possible. Women who wish to avoid pregnancy should obtain the best available contraception for their individual case. There is no evidence that sickle cell disease carries an increased risk of thrombosis in relation to the contraceptive pill. Therefore contraception in women with sickle cell disease can be approached in precisely the same manner as for individuals with normal haemoglobin. In order of preference those methods which appear to be most acceptable to the individuals and also most effective are as follows:

1 Combined low dose oral contraceptive pill.
2 Progesterone only contraceptive pill (a barrier method should be used with this pill)
3 Barrier method (condom and/or diaphragm plus spermicidal cream)
4 Depo-Provera (medroxyprogesterone acetate)

Depo-Provera is an injectable form of progesterone which is given as a single injection into a muscle. The progesterone is then released slowly over a period of about three months. It has the advantage in areas with under-developed health care facilities that a single visit to a clinic or a visit by a medical team can provide three months' contraceptive cover with one injection. It has also been shown in Jamaica that Depo-Provera increases the proportion of fetal haemoglobin in the sickle cells and this reduces slightly the severity and frequency of sickle cell crises. Unfortunately many women suffer significant vaginal bleeding with Depo-Provera and menstruation becomes very erratic. For those women who find the preparation acceptable, however, it is an excellent form of contraception. All the other methods are effective with the main failures being due to the woman omitting to take doses of the contraceptive pill or the couple forgetting to use the barrier method. Those women who are on a contraceptive pill should be treated with subcutaneous heparin during prolonged or particularly severe painful crises involving periods of bed rest longer than two or three days. This is to prevent deep vein thrombosis. There are reasons to avoid using the contraceptive pill in sickle cell disease. These are the same as for any woman: age greater than forty years; cigarette smoker; obesity; previous history of thrombosis.

## TERMINATION OF PREGNANCY

Requests for termination of pregnancy by women with sickle cell disease are uncommon. However, on occasions there are reasons why a woman will be unhappy to be pregnant at that time. In a person with sickle cell disease a termination of pregnancy can be justified because of the risk to the health of the mother. There is also the additional strain of an unwanted child being brought up by a woman who is prone to painful crises.

If termination of pregnancy is to be carried out under a general anaesthetic the same precautions as for other surgery must be taken by medical staff. It will not usually be necessary for the patient to be transfused.

## PREGNANCY

The most important aspect of managing pregnancy is that the pregnancy should be planned and that it should be managed by a co-ordinated team consisting of a haematologist and an obstetrician. Monitoring throughout pregnancy should be offered by the medical team on a regular basis and it is important that the mother attends for her appointments and investigations.

When pregnancy is confirmed counselling may be required particularly if the sickle status of the partner is unknown. Ideally pre-pregnancy counselling will have taken place as part of the long-term management of the patient. It is important that the mother takes folic acid. Iron therapy should be prescribed only if the iron stores are reduced. The monitoring of fetal development using ultrasound is important and if there is any doubt about the baby's progress further investigation may be needed.

The main dilemma of management of pregnancy for doctors at the present time is whether or not to institute a transfusion regime through pregnancy. Over the past five or ten years in the UK there has been a general move towards using blood transfusions in homozygous sickle cell disease pregnancies. However, a recent trial from the United States showed no benefit from blood transfusions and this policy should therefore be reviewed. It will probably remain an individual matter however and those women who are known to be moderately severe sufferers and need three or more admissions to hospital each year on average may still do better on a transfusion regime than without. Mild sickle cell sufferers who are very rarely admitted to hospital may well manage without transfusions. In the past it was common for untransfused patients to require blood transfusions later in pregnancy because of a fall in haemoglobin. Although this is largely due to normal processes, a pregnant woman with a haemoglobin of 4.5–5.0 g/dl needs urgent attention and it is better to avoid this situation if possible. The issue of blood transfusion in pregnancy is discussed in more detail in Chapter 6.

Women with haemoglobin S/haemoglobin C disease (see p. 96) have a fairly normal haemoglobin throughout pregnancy and here the fear is that they may have an increased risk of thrombosis. Pregnancy carries an increased risk of thrombosis, and in Hb S/Hb C disease the sickling cells and high haemoglobin make this worse. It has been recommended that subcutaneous heparin therapy (injections of heparin under the skin) should be used for the final six months of pregnancy. There are no trial data to support this, but it represents a safe and sensible alternative to transfusion therapy.

Regardless of whether the doctors adopt a transfusion regime or not, any sickle cell disease crisis occurring in pregnancy should be dealt with urgently. Adequate hydration must be achieved and maintained rapidly and good pain relief obtained as soon as possible. If the mother is not improving within 48 or 72 hours and has not previously been given exchange blood transfusion this should then be strongly considered.

The management of labour should be undertaken as normal and there are no obvious reasons to exclude any pain-killing drugs or particular ways of managing the pregnancy. However, in an untransfused sickle cell patient the prospect of epidural anaesthesia or a caesarean section are rather more daunting than in the transfused subject. Patients with sickle cell disease are as likely to suffer from high blood pressure as other individuals. Rarely, this can lead to eclampsia late in pregnancy and this must be distinguished from a sickle cell crisis. The pains of labour are usually easy to distinguish from those of crisis; the mother is usually quite clear on this point.

Pain relief in labour usually involves pethidine, preferably given through some device that the patient can control. Nitrous oxide appears to be safe provided oxygen is inhaled with it. The fully transfused sickle cell patient can be managed as normal but in the untransfused patient an anaesthetic for Caesarean section should be administered with very good pre-operative hydration. Oxygen must be given before, during and after delivery. Throughout labour it is of vital importance that good hydration is maintained at all times and in the untransfused patient subcutaneous heparin should be considered following delivery to prevent thrombosis.

Most mothers with sickle cell disease seem to be well supported following the delivery, usually by their extended family. The importance of warm and dry accommodation is obviously paramount at this time and during the pregnancy social service support should have been enlisted to try and ensure optimum conditions for the return home of mother and baby. Obviously if the partner has been tested and found to be a carrier for sickle cell disease, testing of the child for sickle cell disease should be given special attention by medical staff and the result conveyed to the parents as soon as possible.

EIGHT

# Sickle Cell Disease in Childhood

## DIAGNOSIS

Babies with sickle cell disease are born healthy because of the presence of fetal haemoglobin in their blood. Sickle haemoglobin takes over and becomes the dominant haemoglobin by the time they are approximately six months old. Symptoms and problems related to sickle cell disease can commence at any time after three months of age although six to nine months is the most usual. The time at which the diagnosis is made is most important for a number of reasons. First, if the diagnosis is made at birth this enables the parents to be advised about the problems of sickle cell disease. Counselling can be provided about how these problems may affect their family. Second, making the diagnosis at birth enables the initial problems of sickle cell disease to be recognized immediately they occur. Although anxiety will still obviously arise within the family, the reason for the child's illness will be apparent from an early stage and anxiety can be minimized. The parents will be aware of the serious complications of sickle cell disease and will be in a position to seek help rapidly from their general practitioner or a specialist centre, so minimizing sickness and the risk of mortality in the first year of life. In addition, unnecessary investigations into the possible cause of painful episodes of other problems related to sickle cell disease will be avoided. Finally, counselling parents early will enable them to make decisions about further pregnancies in the light of the knowledge that they have at least one child with sickle cell disease. Such counselling can be provided before the onset of another pregnancy. For these reasons it is imperative that the diagnosis is made at birth or as soon afterwards as possible.

## Achieving Early Diagnosis

Testing of the mother at her first antenatal clinic visit should have led to her partner being tested. This will have identified the couple as at risk of having an infant with sickle cell disease. In order to ensure that cases are not overlooked, all infants should be tested for sickle and other haemoglobin disorders at birth as part of the routine screening programmes for phenylketonuria (PKU) and thyroid disease. In areas with very few couples at risk this approach may not be cost effective. If this is the case obstetricians and paediatricians must ensure that any infant who appears to be of an ethnic minority group at risk of sickle cell disease or other haemoglobin disorders is tested. In Jamaica testing is undertaken using cord blood samples but heel prick specimens as for PKU can also be used, as they have been for the last ten years in Birmingham.

# CLINICAL PROBLEMS IN CHILDREN

## Hand–foot Syndrome

This is often the earliest sign of sickle cell disease and is caused by sickling involving the bones and soft tissues of the hands and feet. In England about one per cent of children with sickle cell disease develop this complication. The reason for these areas being at special risk from sickling is not known but it may relate to their being rapidly growing areas of bone tissue. The episode is characterized by the child becoming distressed and by swelling of the hands and feet. This may affect one or all four limbs and there may be loss of function of the affected limb. X-ray examination may show some destruction of bone. Although the condition usually settles down quickly, in severe cases it is important to exclude osteomyelitis by blood cultures and further radiology. The condition is managed by resting the affected limb, maintaining good hydration and using pain relief as for other painful crises.

## Painful Crises

These occur quite frequently in childhood with approximately three per year per child. As for adults, many children will have very few episodes of painful crisis but a few patients may have many such episodes. Severe complicated crises such as chest syndrome and girdle syndrome seem to be less common in children. Management should be as for adult sickle crises including good hydration and exclusion of infection (see Chapter 3).

## Splenic Infarction and Sequestration Crises

Children with sickle cell disease are born with normally functioning spleens, but repeated micro-sickling episodes within the spleen lead to the loss of all spleen function by the age of five years. At this age tests of spleen function might show no function present. There are two important aspects regarding the spleen in children with sickle cell disease. The first is the increased risk of infections from pneumococcus and other bacteria due to the loss of the spleen's filtering function. Children with sickle cell disease should receive penicillin twice daily or, if compliance is thought to be a potential problem, monthly injections of an intramuscular depot penicillin. This is painful, however, and unlikely to be tolerated beyond three years of age. Penicillin effectively prevents episodes of pneumococcal infection in young children with sickle cell disease. Immunization with pneumococcal vaccine may also be useful although on its own it is inadequate to prevent pneumococcal infection.

The second problem is splenic sequestration. Early diagnosis of splenic sequestration can be achieved by parents learning to feel for the spleen (splenic palpation) so that if their child becomes unwell and lethargic they can search for the enlarging spleen by feeling the abdomen. Identification of an enlarging spleen must be followed by immediate attendance at the paediatric ward responsible for care of the child.

## Strokes

Cerebrovascular accidents in sickle cell disease patients are a devastating event that may either be life threatening or lead to permanent brain damage. It is thought that many of the strokes are related to malformations of the blood vessels in the brain since strokes are most common in children with sickle cell disease rather than in adults. Management of the stroke is by exchange blood transfusion. This should be continued for some time although the optimum duration for transfusion therapy has not been established. No controlled trial data exist in favour of this management but it does seem effective in preventing recurrences. It may simply be delaying another stroke until the transfusion regime is stopped.

## Bed Wetting

As discussed in Chapter 4 the inability of the kidney to concentrate urine is due to damage to the kidney tubules from the sickling of blood in the renal medulla. This leads to increased bed wetting in children and adolescents with sickle cell disease. It is doubtful whether any treatment is helpful other than lifting in the night or alarm bells. Often, the family knowing that bed wetting is common in sickle cell disease because of the effect on the kidneys is sufficient to remove much of the anxiety, embarrassment and annoyance associated with bed wetting.

## Leg Ulcers

Leg ulcers are uncommon in children in the UK although in Jamaica and Africa they are a very common and disruptive complication. They are particularly problematic because of the loss of schooling. Management has been discussed in Chapter 4.

## Immunization of Children with Sickle Cell Disease

Children with sickle cell disease should receive all normal immunizations. Indeed it is particularly important that they should do so since their immunological response to some infections may be reduced. In addition to covering against whooping cough, diphtheria, tetanus, polio, rubella, mumps and measles they should receive penicillin as a preventive treatment against pneumococcal infections, and possibly a pneumococcal vaccine as well (see above).

## COUNSELLING FOR PARENTS OF CHILDREN WITH SICKLE CELL DISEASE

The parents of children with sickle cell disease require a lot of support and advice in addition to counselling. Factual advice needs to cover aspects such as crisis management, immunization, spleen palpation and practical decisions about the care of other children when the affected child is in hospital or unwell. They may need advice about suitable footwear to reduce the risk of leg ulcers and of the possible occurrence of bed wetting persisting later into childhood than with other more healthy children. They may require counselling regarding future pregnancies and with regard to their own feelings of guilt about having produced a child with an illness. There is also the possibility that they may harbour negative feelings towards the child.

Before the child has become unwell the parents and child should meet the consultant responsible for the care of the child and also the ward sister in charge of the ward to which children are admitted. If there are sickle cell counselling facilities available they should be introduced to the sickle cell counsellor and possibly to the self-help groups locally. Because some children with sickle cell disease are only mildly affected, parents should not feel that the child is an invalid or needs to be managed as such. The continuing care and attention of brothers and sisters should also be emphasized so that their schooling or emotional development does not suffer.

## DEVELOPMENTAL MILESTONES

There is no obvious reason why developmental milestones should not be completely normal for a child with sickle cell disease.

However, it is likely that in the more severely affected child some of these milestones may be delayed because of episodes of illness or admissions to hospital. Psychological development may also suffer because of such traumas. There is also some evidence to suggest that physical growth in the early stages is retarded in individuals with sickle cell disease and that they enter puberty and menarche late. However, there does not appear to be any good evidence to suggest that final height attained is any less than their normal peers and indeed the so-called typical sickle cell image is of a tall, slim person. Clearly with a child prone to recurrent episodes of ill health interspersed with periods of good health close attention should be paid to achieving developmental milestones. This should be achieved by attending a clinic with a paediatrician or preferably a paediatric haematologist with special interest and expertise in sickle cell disease. Access to hospital should be free and open. Good relations with the general practitioner must be encouraged, but it should be possible for parents to bring their child directly to the ward or relevant area on their own initiative if necessary. On arrival they should be met by staff who are skilled in caring for children with sickle cell disease and a doctor who has similar expertise should be available. Obviously, if a child is admitted to hospital with a painful crisis it will not be possible for at least the first few days to attend to any educational matters. But certainly for admissions of longer than four or five days, and where severe pain is not involved, then continuing education must be a very high priority. This is particularly true for those few children who will spend prolonged periods of time in hospital and have numerous admissions. Similarly, facilities for a parent to stay in hospital with the child should also be provided and encouraged while bearing in mind the requirements of other children at home.

## SCHOOLING

People with sickle cell disease are unlikely to be able to earn their living in the long term by physical labour. It is therefore essential that their education is maintained and that their academic potential is maximized. Their ability to find employment after leaving school should be as good as it would have been had they not had sickle cell disease. A number of aspects need to be in place before this can be achieved. First, the parents need to be well advised regarding the problems of sickle cell disease and the possible effect on their child's education should they suffer multiple crises. It is probably only the parents who can ensure that the child's education is continuing if episodes of schooling are punctuated by periods of time in hospital. Second, as mentioned above, hospitals need to be able to provide educational facilities for children. These should be available not just for those children who are in hospital for a long time but also those children who require frequent short admissions for example with painful crises. Third, school teachers need to be informed about the consequences of sickle cell disease on the child and the school itself needs to be prepared to provide additional schooling for the child as appropriate. Sickle cell disease should be seen as a condition with a potential for jeopardizing the success of the education process for the child and not as a disruption to class. Resources should be mobilized to continue the child's education. With the agreement of the family, the consultant responsible for the child's care should make available to the school information about sickle cell disease. Once the school is appropriately informed about the nature of sickle cell disease and how it can affect children, it can make arrangements to ensure minimum disruption to the child's education.

NINE

# Community Care

Many patients with sickle cell disease are very well and fit and healthy in between sickle cell crises. Many patients have only occasional sickle cell crises or other acute problems. However there is a significant minority of patients for whom sickle cell disease is a severe chronic disabling condition because of complications of the illness. In order to prevent, or help to prevent, sickle cell painful crises and other complications such as infections, it is important that patients have good accommodation and social circumstances – at least as far as is possible. For these reasons the care of individuals with sickle cell disease must extend into the community and take account of domestic, employment and educational issues. Community care is particularly important in relation to the chronic medical and social problems related to the condition, advice regarding social security benefits and allowances, and also education. The organization and co-ordination of services for sickle cell disease should be based upon a Sickle Cell Centre and work as a group as shown in Fig. 4. This diagram presents a suggestion for the organization of total care for sickle cell disease patients.

## CHRONIC PROBLEMS

Individuals with sickle cell disease suffer disruption in education and employment and these are likely to put strains upon their financial resources. They may require improved accommodation. Counsellors and health advisers are needed to discuss education and employment problems with teachers and employers. As Sickle Cell Centres develop and funding is provided it will be important to

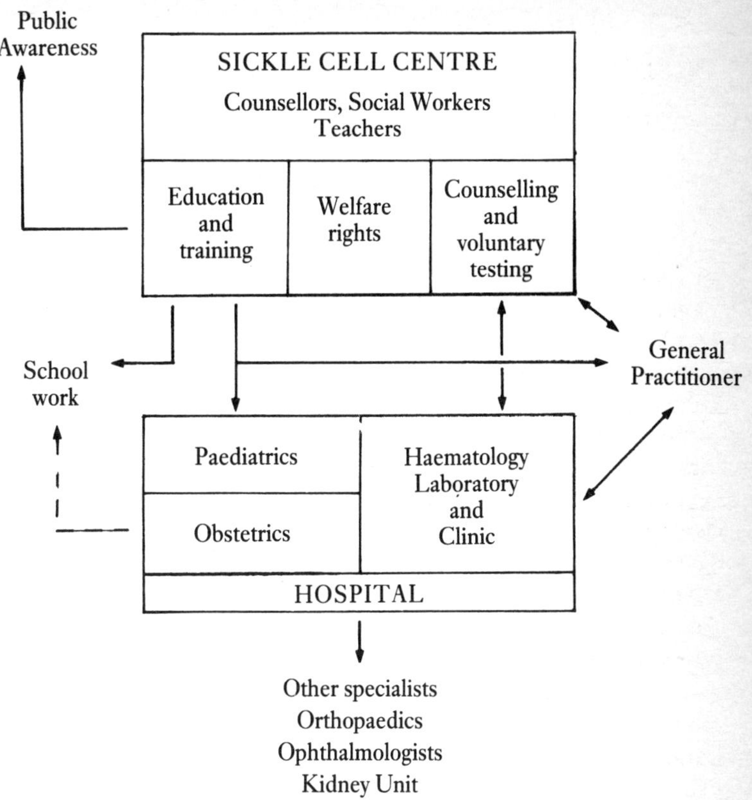


Care should be co-ordinated by:
- Head of Sickle Cell Centre
- Consultant (chairperson of local group)
- Social Worker
- Counsellor
- GP representative
- Patient's representative (e.g. OSCAR, SCS)

**Fig. 4** Model for care of sickle cell disease

address these issues. This will require co-ordination between the counsellor or health adviser, social worker and medical staff. Ideally, a Sickle Cell Centre would include a welfare rights expert.

Physical problems such as chronic pain, pregnancy, leg ulcers and problems with joints may all require specific assistance at home both from medical practitioners and from nurses and health advisers. This may include alterations to accommodation and input from occupational therapists. The care of children at home, either in the case of a mother with sickle cell disease or in the case of children having the disease, may also require special skills and input from health visitors and other health advisers.

All of these issues may require the availability of in-depth expertise about community issues relating to sickle cell disease. Although each health professional involved with a person with sickle cell disease may not have to be an expert in the subject, it is important to have a core of experts who can co-ordinate and educate and train other health care professionals in the management of sickle cell disease.

## BENEFITS

People with sickle cell disease are eligible to apply for registration as disabled. This opens the way to a large range of benefits but also carries the risk of stigmatization and may impose substantial limitations on the ability of the person to find employment other than in certain sheltered areas of work. The decision as to whether disabled status should be sought should follow discussions between the individual and his or her health advisers so that the advantages and disadvantages of disabled status can be assessed. Mobility allowances are an important benefit for people with sickle cell disease to claim. It is important that patients should be mobile and able to attend the clinics without exposing themselves to long periods of standing in the cold at bus stops. Damaged joints will be protected from further injury if the need to walk long distances is removed.

## EDUCATION

This can be divided into education of the general public, teachers, employers and the education of health care professionals. All levels of health care workers require education about sickle cell disease, from doctors to meals-on-wheels assistants. Lack of knowledge of sickle cell disease is caused by a number of factors which are discussed in more detail in Chapter 11. Many black people live in identifiable areas and attend a limited number of medical practices. It should therefore be possible in the initial phases to target this education to those medical practices, social workers and other health care workers who are most likely to come into contact with persons with sickle cell disease. Eventually such education, on perhaps a broader level, should be extended nationwide.

Similarly the education of teachers and employers about the disease is more likely to succeed by specific targeting of schools and workplaces where individuals with sickle cell disease are known to attend. It appears unreasonable to expect teachers to have an awareness of all the various disorders which may affect the children they teach. However, with the consent of parents and children it should be feasible to provide educational packages and interviews with teachers who are directly involved with the care of people with sickle cell disease. In this way, a more understanding attitude towards occasional absences from school or work should be engendered.

Education of the general public has so far been tackled only on a very limited basis. There seem to be a number of reasons for this including a lack of funds, a lack of a co-ordinated view of what would be required in such education and the fear that major public educational programmes could result in racially motivated attacks from groups of the white population. One other problem with large-scale education of the public is that it is probable that a well-organized campaign would generate a large number of enquiries for further information and advice about sickle cell disease. It is therefore important that before any such large-scale public education programme takes place, education of health care professionals should be undertaken and specific advice services available.

## A MODEL FOR COMMUNITY CARE IN SICKLE CELL DISEASE

There are a number of features that should apply to the ideal support system for individuals with sickle cell disease. First, there should be good liaison between the hospital and community carers. In this context community carers should include the general practitioner, the patient and their family, sickle cell counsellors and other health care workers. Such a scheme implies that a second requirement of a good community service system would be education of health care professionals regarding sickle cell disease. This education should be appropriate to the individuals concerned and would therefore have to be presented differently to medical practitioners, social workers, health visitors and home attendants. Third, the patients themselves must have access to good counselling support and be fully educated in their knowledge of sickle cell disease. In this way, should there have been any failure in the education of health care professionals the patient will be able to correct any misapprehensions.

The fourth point is that there should be a community education programme. This should be aimed initially at the black population, but in a defined time span be extended to the community at large. This should be developed in parallel with the fifth item of community care which should involve a testing programme for individuals who wish to be tested for the sickle cell trait. Again a good testing programme must be supported with adequate counselling, and back up support facilities and education of health care workers in the community.

Sixth, there is a requirement for targeted educational programmes aimed at the schools and the workplace. Finally these should be co-ordinated by a multidisciplinary steering group (see Fig. 4).

## REQUIREMENTS FOR SICKLE CELL COMMUNITY CARE

In broad terms there is an association between the number of individuals with sickle cell disease and the number of people with sickle cell trait and people who may have the trait. From this it is possible to estimate approximately how many community workers are required. One sickle cell counsellor/social worker should be able to cope with approximately thirty patients with sickle cell disease and to cover all the other aspects relating to their management. This means one counsellor for every 5000–10000 of the at risk population. In addition to providing specific education and counselling to these sufferers, many of whom will be only mildly affected, the community worker should be able to develop educational programmes for the community, targeted educational programmes for doctors, nurses, teachers and employers, and develop liaison between the hospital and the home. Individual workers will develop specialist interests as their number increases. In other words if there are three or four sickle cell counsellors it is likely that one of these would be a trained social worker and another would have a major interest in educational issues. All would need to have good counselling and communication skills and have a sound knowledge of the medical problems.

Secretarial support is also important and each worker needs the support of one-third to one-half of a secretary. Accommodation is required to provide facilities for taking blood samples within the centre and also a walk-in advice system. From previous work carried out in Birmingham, counselling and additional testing sessions in general practices and other community centres are also popular. All these arrangements should lead to an improved level of education of both patients and the general community about sickle cell disease. An improved awareness of their own problems by the patients themselves, together with education of teachers and employers, should improve the general health of sickle cell suffers and their employment and educational records. Such a service clearly needs to be funded from Department of Health funds, perhaps supported by some social security revenue. In this way the continuation of such services can be assured. There is no doubt that once set up the level of need shown will be substantially greater than was originally perceived.

Some of the services described above could be provided by self-help groups such as OSCAR (Organization for Sickle Cell Anaemia Research) and the Sickle Cell Society. But if this is the case it is important that there should be adequate monitoring of the medical content of advice and support given. The services should also be clearly contracted to the self-help group so that funding of the services is assured in the long term. These aspects will be developed further in Chapter 11.

TEN

# Hospital Services

Inadequate hospital services are probably the most frequent complaint of patients with sickle cell disease. The requirements for support in hospital usually come at a time of very great need. The patients are in positions of great dependence due to severe pain or other illness and find it difficult at that time to articulate their needs. However, unfortunate experiences are remembered and can lead to major problems of confidence between the health workers and the individual patients. Bad experiences may often be relayed to the sickle cell community at large, thereby further damaging relationships between the community of people with sickle cell disease and their families and the hospital which is attempting to provide care for them. Such problems are exacerbated when, as is usually the case in the UK, the great majority of health care professionals are white and the majority of patients are black.

The issues of race in the provision of health care have been examined by others in the field of sickle cell disease. It often appears that on those occasions when good communications, trust and confidence are most required between the sufferer and the carers this relationship is jeopardized by an atmosphere of fear, anxiety and uncertainty on behalf of the sufferer. This is associated with a lack of comprehension and often a similar feeling of fear and uncertainty and distrust on behalf of the carers. It will be of little avail if the material aspects and practical matters of caring for patients with sickle cell disease in hospital are in place, if an appropriate atmosphere of mutual trust, understanding and consideration is not present. Education is paramount in this regard both in the provision of optimal care to patients in hospital and in the liaison between hospital and the community.

This education extends both to the health care professionals and to the patients themselves. The patients need to be fully aware of the nature of their condition, of why they suffer the symptoms and problems that they do, and why doctors and nurses have to conform to certain procedures when they are admitted to hospital. It is only then that the sickle cell sufferer will come to feel confident and understand the role of health care professionals within the hospital environment.

Similarly it is of the utmost importance that the doctors, nurses and other health professionals are knowledgeable about sickle cell disease and know the problems that the individual sufferer may have had to deal with. In addition to being aware of the medical aspects of sickle cell disease hospitals should also be aware of the cultural requirements of patients regarding differences in nursing care and diet. Most hospital catering departments are aware of the dietary needs of Asian groups and vegetarians but so far little attention has been paid to the dietary requirements of Afro-Caribbeans. Many of these requirements are easily met and require very little effort on behalf of hospital staff. But making this effort would actually make a great deal of difference to the atmosphere developed for the patient and would help to engender an atmosphere of confidence. This might lead to an alleviation of anxiety and therefore help symptoms in an indirect way.

## PRACTICAL ASPECTS FOR MANAGEMENT OF SICKLE CELL DISEASE IN HOSPITAL

A hospital practice of between thirty and forty individuals with homozygous sickle cell disease would expect to utilize two or three hospital beds on a fairly regular basis. Hospital managers should therefore be aware of the bed requirements of their local population of sickle cell disease sufferers and allocate beds, nurses and other resources appropriately.

In most districts patients with sickle cell disease will be managed by a haematologist and in general this is a desirable state of affairs. However, in some districts there may well be a consultant physician with a particular interest in sickle cell disease and in such an instance it would be completely appropriate that such an individual should take charge of sickle cell patients. However, if this is the case then such a physician should be responsible for all the sickle cell sufferers attending regularly at that hospital so that all cases are seen by either an individual consultant or a single department. Only in this way will a body of medical and nursing expertise be built in one particular area. Specific junior doctors can then be targeted with regard to training in aspects of sickle cell disease. A system where sickle cell patients are looked after by a wide variety of consultant physicians and haematologists throughout one particular district is to be avoided and such districts should develop a policy of management of sickle cell disease that concentrates their care in one unit.

Thus the ideal situation would be that all the sickle cell sufferers would be looked after by either one physician–haematologist or one or two doctors working together. When they are admitted to hospital they should go to a single ward or single pair of male and female wards so that expertise is concentrated in that area.

It is also very important that direct admission to this area is available both by the patients themselves contacting the ward or doctor on call directly. Alternatively if the initial contact is to the general practitioner, the general practitioner should be able to admit directly to this area following a brief telephone call to the doctor on call for sickle cell disease. This should be a 24 hour, 365 day a year service. Clearly there will not always be doctors specifically for looking after sickle cell disease patients but ideally these doctors should be looking after other haematological problems related to that area. Under no circumstances should waiting around in accident, emergency or casualty departments by individuals known to have sickle cell disease be tolerated. Once patients are admitted it is very important that they are attended to promptly by doctors who are expert in or at least are familiar with the problems of sickle cell disease. Only in this way can surgical and other medical emergencies be promptly and rapidly excluded so that the patient can be given adequate pain relief. Obviously this is very straightforward if the pain is localized to the limbs or the back but occasionally abdominal pains or chest pains are present and obviously on such occasions it is important to exclude other complicating disorders such as gall-stones, appendicitis, perforated ulcers that may require surgical intervention and also other medical conditions such as heart attacks, myocardial infarctions and pulmonary emboli.

Liaison with the Community Sickle Cell Service is also of great importance. This can be mobilized to provide an education service for nursing and medical staff in hospital. The same message is put across to the patients and health workers to provide them with a fully integrated comprehensive sickle cell service.

The outpatient department also has a major role to play in the management of sickle cell disease. On a relatively superficial but important level it provides a meeting place for patients which can improve the sufferers' morale. Because doctors and nurses are aware that individual sufferers meet together on a regular basis in the waiting room for clinics this also helps to keep the carers alert in the knowledge that any adverse stories will be passed around. Patients with severe sickle cell disease may need to be seen every three months, whereas mild sufferers will need only an annual review.

A regular specific clinic for sickle cell disease provides a number of advantages for the medical and nursing staff. A practice of thirty or forty homozygous sickle cell disease patients should provide plenty of work for a monthly sickle cell clinic when most of the routine problems can be dealt with. Patients should of course be aware that they can be seen at any clinic should they ring up beforehand. Obviously when numbers increase to fifty or sixty patients with homozygous sickle cell disease it may be appropriate to run a weekly clinic with specific medical and nursing staff in attendance. Seeing a succession of individuals with sickle cell disease does make it much easier for the doctors to address the specific management issues related to sickle cell disease rather than mixing up these patients with other anaemias and leukaemias. Doctors can discuss in a systematic manner the issues of appropriate accommodation, contraception, prevention of leg ulcers, general attention to good health and prevention of sickle cell crises. They will also have time to address other aspects of health education regarding the planning of pregnancies, screening for development of gall-stones, eye clinic follow-ups and advice about maintaining their health in the 'steady state'.

## MANAGEMENT OF THE STEADY STATE

The steady state in sickle cell disease is a jargon term used to describe the state of well being of patients between sickle cell crises when they are also free of other complications such as leg ulcers.

Maintaining patients in the steady state is the current aim of therapy and also most experimental ideas for treatment in the future.

At the present time there are certain points that we do know that may well help maintain people within the steady state. An attention to the environment in which the person lives is important. They should have dry, warm accommodation and ideally should not be required to walk long distances in the cold or to wait around cold bus stops in the winter. All of these could precipitate sickle cell crises.

It is also important that they drink a good amount of fluid, at least 3–4 pints each day, to make sure they do not get dry. If they start to feel any painful episodes then they should increase the amount of fluid that they drink. Since alcohol can have a dehydrating effect and thus produce risks of precipitating sickle cell crisis it is important that people with sickle cell disease are counselled about the effect of alcohol and that they moderate their use of this drug.

Protection to ankles and prevention of leg ulcers can be made by appropriate footwear and also by elevating the feet when they are not walking around, i.e. by putting their feet on a stool.

Prevention of infection is also important and for this reason penicillin 250 mg twice a day will help prevent life-threatening infections due to the pneumococcal bacteria. Medical advice should be sought promptly should any temperature of illness become apparent. Taking folic acid will certainly prevent folic acid deficiency and anaemia due to lack of this vitamin, but there is not very good evidence to suggest that anaemia due to folic acid deficiency is common in sickle cell disease.

## Folic acid

This vitamin is important for the production of haemoglobin in the red cells. Occasionally in people who have a very poor diet, low in green vegetables and other fresh foods, folic acid deficiency can occur and anaemia be the result. Because in sickle cell disease the bone marrow has to work very hard to keep up with the production of haemoglobin a good supply of folic acid is particularly important. It is quite usual for folic acid to be prescribed on a regular basis such as 5 mg a day. In fact this is quite a high dose and although it does not cause any toxic effects 5 mg once a week is probably more than adequate. There is very little evidence to support the idea that patients with sickle cell disease get into major trouble if they do not take folic acid but the usual practice is to recommend its use.

## Penicillin

Penicillin has been shown to reduce or even prevent the risk of infections caused by the pneumococcal bacteria in childhood. Although good studies have not been carried out it is likely that continuing to take penicillin will prevent infections from this organism in adults as well. In patients who have had their spleen removed because of injuries to it in road accidents or because it has been removed in the course of other treatment, it is known that there is a small but important risk of infections with pneumococcus that can continue for some time. Since patients with sickle cell disease have no functional spleen because of sickling within the organ they are also at risk from pneumococcal infections. It is therefore advisable that patients with sickle cell disease should take penicillin 250 mg twice a day to prevent pneumococcal infections. How long this prophylaxis treatment should continue is a matter of much debate. A case can certainly be made for continuing life-long since the risk, although small, does persist. As people get older they tend to live in smaller groups as they settle down and have a family. This makes them less likely to be exposed to pneumococcal infections than when for instance they are at school or college. For this reason it has often been stated that individuals can stop taking the penicillin when they reach their early 20s. However there is no scientific basis for this and it is merely a feeling. Certainly patients often do not like to continue taking medication on a life-long basis and this makes the decision even more difficult to make. In the ideal world the taking of penicillin on a regular basis is to be recommended. Whether this is appropriate for the individual patient however needs to be discussed between the medical team caring for them and the person themselves.

## RESEARCH

Sickle cell disease has proved a frustrating disorder to research but sickle cell sufferers themselves and their organized bodies are very keen to see research continuing. The community of sickle cell sufferers usually provides an excellent group of individuals from which to recruit subjects for research projects that have received the approval of local ethical committees. Research activity associated with outpatient clinic, inpatient hospital ward and the community are very valuable in demonstrating a commitment to the disorder. Commitment by research workers in the field is readily transmitted to the sufferers and leads to a dramatic improvement in morale. If the research workers are involved with patients when they are admitted and come and visit them both for social reasons and also to take samples, this leads to an appreciation by the patients that the medical and nursing staff do have a long-term commitment to sickle cell disease. This will demonstrate that health workers are as keen as the patients to see a useful and realistic treatment for the condition.

ELEVEN

# Self-Help Groups

The development of comprehensive services for patients with sickle cell disease is in its infancy in most parts of the UK. Even in those centres where the needs of sufferers have been recognized for many years the fact that the incidence of the disorder is increasing significantly means that it is difficult to keep pace with the demands. The difficulty of providing adequate facilities for support of sufferers from sickle cell disease and the associated community is not unique to this disorder. It is also found in other conditions such as haemophilia, cystic fibrosis and leukaemias. In all these conditions the facilities for acute care are usually well established, but there are additional needs, and self-help groups have developed in order to fill the gaps. They also act as pressure groups to improve facilities and often raise money. However, there are special features related to sickle cell disease which make self-help groups particularly important.

1 Sickle cell disease is a relatively new disorder in the UK growing at a much faster rate than the existing resources. It is probable that the current resources are about ten years behind those required.
2 Inequalities in health care affect the black community in particular and lead to a tendency for under provision and also lack of update of existing services.
3 Most doctors, hospital managers and ancillary staff in positions of authority probably trained more than fifteen years ago. They would not have been fully trained or educated about the medical or social problems of sickle cell disease and certainly not about the needs of sufferers.

In the UK there has been no directive from the Department of Health to District Health Authorities to require them to produce services and facilities to sickle cell sufferers. It has, in the main, fallen to hospital doctors to plead the case of the patients and the need for resources to district or regional health managers. Although it is often possible to gain small sums of money, all too often doctors are perceived as empire building or pleading on their own behalf. They become less effective in achieving additional funding, unless the message can be reinforced in great detail by the provision of hard data. If this situation is to improve, pressure will need to come from the community.

## ROLE OF SELF-HELP GROUPS

There are a number of clear roles that any self-help group in any disorder should be working towards.

1. They should make strong representations to the Department of Health and Health Service Managers to raise awareness at all levels.
2. They should provide support to patients with informal counselling, advice services or centres, holiday homes, hostels and possibly social centres.
3. Service provision. It may be appropriate on occasions for self-help groups to provide services that would normally be the function of Health Authorities. These might include testing of individuals for sickle cell trait status, education of the public and even more formal counselling and advice systems. However, if these are conducted on an ad hoc basis by self-help groups, funding tends to lapse after a period. It is therefore important that such service provision is undertaken on a contract basis from Health Authorities so that funding for these services is guaranteed. It is very easy for self-help groups to fall into the trap of providing essential services to the Health Service which, after a period of years, become established by custom and which Health Authorities then refuse to continue.

In this way Health Authorities can escape their obligations to patients and receive large subsidies from the voluntary sector.

4 Research support. There is also a need to raise funds to support research. This is particularly difficult for the black community which tends to be poor with a larger proportion of unemployed members than the population as a whole. Large efforts are being made to raise awareness and funds for sickle cell disease, however. Continuity of income over the long term is important. This would enable activities to be planned in advance. Medical research is very expensive and even a quite modest programme of research may cost £50 000–£100 000 a year.

Certainly there is a great need for the voluntary bodies to work together with the hospitals to improve liaison between the community and the hospital. This would be to the benefit of patients but also for education of the community at large. An active self-help group should act as a ginger group to impress the importance of services for sickle cell disease on holders of hospital budgets and those people who have responsibilities for the development of health care policies. In this way the self-help group can act both as a stimulus to the development of improved services and, once services are provided, as a patient advocate to ensure that the service standards are maintained. One of the difficulties of self-help groups acting as the providers of services is that their watchdog function is compromised.

## CONCLUSION

Services for sickle cell disease, although improving, are lagging behind the numbers of cases arising in the UK. Major obstacles to progress are the inadequate education of health care professionals, disadvantage within the black community and institutionalized racism. It is unlikely that services will be improved unless there is a very vigorous and active co-operation between those providing services for patients and the self-help groups in lobbying budget holders and health care policy makers.

TWELVE

# Will There Be a Cure?

It is now over forty years since the abnormal haemoglobin was first recognized and yet in terms of a specific cure or treatment for sickle cell disease things are really very little further forward. What has happened in that time has been a massive investment of money, time and effort on behalf of researchers, mainly in the USA, towards finding a cure. One of the difficulties in sickle cell disease is the sheer number of abnormal haemoglobin molecules present within the body's red cells. In order to change the molecule millions and millions of haemoglobin molecules would have to be altered and many potential drugs also react with other proteins and cause unacceptable side effects. One of the first, and most promising, examples of such a drug was cyanate. This reacted with one end of the haemoglobin molecule and was moderately effective in reducing the amount of sickling. Unfortunately it also tended to bind to the end of a number of other protein molecules, particularly in the eye and in the nerves. This caused unacceptable side effects such as cataracts in the eyes and weakness and numbness in the legs due to nerve damage. Many other agents have also been investigated and discarded because of this potential for side effects.

It can be helpful to look at the ways in which the disorder might be treated if it were possiblc to do so. These can be divided into various groups.

1 Alter the genes – this can work on an individual basis or even on a family or community level.
2 Change the expression of the genes. This would involve switching the production of sickle type haemoglobin to, for example, fetal haemoglobin which does not sickle.

3 Alter the haemoglobin S.
4 Change the secondary effects such as the progressive damage to the red blood cell membrane and the flow properties of the blood.

## ALTERING THE GENES

To alter the genes of an individual would involve a technical feat of genetic engineering. At the present time these techniques are not applicable to humans but only work in micro-organisms such as bacteria. Until the factors controlling the genes are understood it appears unlikely that it will be possible simply to replace normal haemoglobin genes for the haemoglobin S genes.

It has been estimated that, in the absence of malaria to give a selective advantage to the sickle cell trait state, sickle cell disease will die out after about 200–300 years. Obviously this is not of much benefit to sufferers at the present time. In some communities where the severe type of beta thalassaemia is present communities have themselves decided to work towards reducing the incidence of thalassaemia by discouraging couples who both have thalassaemia trait from having children. An alternative is to offer antenatal diagnosis to couples so that they can choose whether or not to continue a pregnancy that is at risk.

Replacing the patient's bone marrow is another way of changing genes. This has generally been considered to be much too drastic to carry out on people with sickle cell disease although it has been attempted in a few individuals with moderate success. Bone marrow transplantation is hazardous to the individual and expensive and is never going to be a useful treatment in tackling the problem of sickle cell disease worldwide.

## CHANGING THE EXPRESSION OF GENES

The possibility of switching the synthesis of sickle haemoglobin back to the fetal haemoglobin that occurs before the baby is born has been investigated for many years. A number of agents have been shown to increase slightly the amount of fetal haemoglobin that is produced because of chemical reactions produced on the DNA, the genetic source material. These drugs are Depo-Provera, a progesterone which is quite useful in contraception, and hydroxyurea which is a cytotoxic drug. This has numerous toxic side effects which make it unsuitable for long-term use in sickle cell disease. It may be that other techniques of a less toxic nature may be discovered that would help in switching on the fetal haemoglobin genes. Again it seems unlikely that there will be any major breakthrough in the next five years. Trying to tackle the problem of gene switching is quite attractive because the number of molecules that must be affected is much less than in trying to react with the sickle haemoglobin after it has been produced.

## CHANGING THE SICKLE HAEMOGLOBIN

The strategies that have been used for changing the sickle haemoglobin have aimed at reacting the protein molecule with other smaller molecules which change its characteristics. Two sites on the sickle haemoglobin are important; one involves the binding of oxygen. If the ability of sickle haemoglobin to bind oxygen could be increased then the number of oxygenating molecules in the red cell would be high and sickling would be less. This can be done for short periods of time with a drug known as BW12C. This has been given in moderate doses to volunteers and is able to change the oxygen-binding characteristics of the sickle haemoglobin. At the present time it has not been used for prolonged periods of time. One of the difficulties with drugs like this is that they encourage the sickle haemoglobin to hold on to the oxygen. The tissues then react by producing a hormone called erythropoietin which encourages the bone marrow to produce more red ells. The decreased sickling would lead to reduced amounts of red cell destruction and the haemoglobin level would increase dramatically. This could lead to life-threatening sickling problems if the drug was suddenly stopped. Drugs meant to alter the oxygen-binding characteristics are less likely to bind to other protein molecules, but this may still be a problem with long-term usage.

Drugs may also be used to block the binding sites in the sickle cell polymer but these have not proved to be safe to use in humans.

## CHANGING SECONDARY EFFECTS

Some drugs have been used to protect the red cell membrane from the damage caused to it by the repeated sickling and unsickling. Some of these are quite effective at reducing damage and sickling in the laboratory but so far there have not been any convincing long-term trials to suggest that any of these agents might be helpful. However, in the short term it is most likely that small benefits might well come from a combination of agents that work in this way and so lead to a reduction in the red cell destruction and an improvement in the flow of blood through the capillaries. Work on these areas is continuing at the present time.

## WORK FOR THE FUTURE

Work will continue along the lines described above. Genetic engineering will lay particular emphasis on trying to understand the switching of the fetal to sickle haemoglobin and trying to get it to go back the other way. It will be important to look at why some patients are much more severely affected than others even when their blood appears to be the same. If it were possible to identify specific reasons why some patients are mildly affected then perhaps these reasons could be manipulated in more severe patients to their own benefit. In the meantime it is important that research and clinical workers do not lose sight of the improvements in care that can be provided to people with sickle cell disease by the universal application of knowledge that is already available regarding prevention of infection, prevention of dehydration and the provision of good access to hospital care. As with so many diseases much suffering that continues at the present time could be helped or alleviated simply by applying the knowledge currently available while waiting and hoping that a cure will not be long coming.

# Appendix: Haemoglobin

In all parts of the world the usual type of haemoglobin present in the red cells of people is called haemoglobin A. In adults this represents over 95 per cent of haemoglobin in the red cells with less than 1 per cent consisting of a different type of haemoglobin called fetal haemoglobin (Hb F) and less than 4 per cent of another haemoglobin known as haemoglobin $A_2$. The usual haemoglobin level in the UK varies from person to person but is usually between 12 and 15 g/dl.

## FETAL HAEMOGLOBIN

This is, as its name suggests, the main type of haemoglobin present in unborn children in the uterus. At the time of birth the type of haemoglobin produced changes from fetal haemoglobin to haemoglobin A. It is thought that unborn babies have fetal haemoglobin because this takes up oxygen more readily than adult haemoglobin A and therefore the baby can take up oxygen from the mother. The factors controlling the switch from fetal to adult haemoglobin are not well understood, despite a great deal of work by scientists. There has been an enormous amount of interest in trying to get adult patients to continue to produce fetal haemoglobin since, if this continued to be produced instead of switching to the adult type, diseases which result from abnormalities of adult type haemoglobin such as sickle cell disease and thalassaemia could be successfully treated. Unfortunately this is proving to be extremely difficult and there does not appear to be any likelihood of major progress in the near future.

In some individuals, again usually from areas where malaria is common but also in Europeans, fetal haemoglobin is produced in increased proportions into adult life. Sometimes this is associated with thalassaemia but not always. Most of these conditions are completely harmless and are simply an incidental and interesting finding. In some patients with sickle cell disease however the persistence of high levels of fetal haemoglobin into adult life does actually lead to a reduced severity. Most individuals with sickle cell disease produce increased amounts of fetal haemoglobin but this is not usually sufficient to reduce the severity of their disease. Until about 15–20 per cent haemoglobin F is reached no change in the severity of sickle cell disease can be expected.

## HAEMOGLOBIN $A_2$

This is always a minor component of the body's haemoglobin and would be completely insignificant if it was not for the fact that in cases of beta thalassaemia the production of haemoglobin $A_2$ is increased. Therefore measuring haemoglobin $A_2$ levels is a useful and important diagnostic test for carriers of beta thalassaemia trait.

## HAEMOGLOBIN S; SICKLE HAEMOGLOBIN; Hb S

These all mean the same thing, namely haemoglobin in which one of the amino acids in the usual haemoglobin A has changed. The particular amino acid involved is the sixth one on the beta chain, which in haemoglobin A is a glutamic acid but in sickle haemoglobin it is a valine.

## SICKLE CELL TRAIT; SICKLE CELL CARRIER

These terms means the same thing, that these people have haemoglobin A and haemoglobin S in their blood with slightly more haemoglobin A than S (Hb S always less than 50 per cent of the total). They can pass on sickle cell haemoglobin on average to half of their children but cannot by themselves pass on sickle cell disease. The sickle cell trait or carrier does not have sickle cell disease.

## HAEMOGLOBIN C

This is another haemoglobin variant at which the sixth amino acid of the beta chain is lysine instead of glutamic acid. This is inherited in the same way as haemoglobin S, is also an antimalarial strategy but produces a less mild clinical disorder than sickle cell disease.

## HAEMOGLOBIN S/BETA THALASSAEMIA

These individuals have inherited a sickle cell haemoglobin gene from one parent and a beta thalassaemia from another. They tend to have sickle cell disease which is as serious as homozygous SS disease and with similar low haemoglobin levels.

## 'HAVING SICKLE'

This term is quite often used and is unhelpful. It does not clearly differentiate between those with sickle cell disease and healthy carriers. It is a confusing term and best avoided.

## RETICULOCYTES

These are young red cells formed less than two days previously. They are called after the network ('reticulum') of protein producing material that can be seen on special blood film stains. Because the bone marrow is producing increased numbers of red cells in sickle cell disease the numbers of reticulocytes in the blood is increased. Measuring the reticulocytes can give a good guide as to the activity of the bone marrow and whether it is coping with the heavy demands made upon it by the haemolytic anaemia.

## STEADY STATE

This is the term used to describe the condition of people with sickle cell disease when they are symptom free. Most studies on sickle cell blood is carried out in the steady state to avoid any effects of a painful crisis or other complication confusing the results. Treatment that would prevent the painful crises would maintain the person in the steady state. This could be of great benefit although the patient would not be 'cured'.

## THALASSAEMIA

There are two types, the beta which affects the beta globin genes and the alpha which affects the alpha globin genes. Beta thalassaemia can interact with sickle haemoglobin to produce a type of sickle cell disease. Alpha thalassaemia can interact with individuals with sickle cell disease to produce a less severe form.

## SICKLE CELL DISEASE

This term has come to embrace all those sickle cell disorders which have symptoms and produce a clinical disorder. The term includes homozygous SS disease, haemoglobin S/haemoglobin C disease, haemoglobin S/beta thalassaemia.

## SICKLE CELL ANAEMIA

This term relates to the fact that patients with sickle cell disease also tend to have anaemia although this is not an essential prerequisite.

Like the term sickle cell disease it tends to be used loosely and does not refer to a specific type.

## HOMOZYGOUS SS DISEASE

This term is rather cumbersome but has the advantage that it is precise, meaning that the person has only haemoglobin S in their blood and no haemoglobin A or thalassaemia. The level of haemoglobin in the blood is usually between 6 and 9 grams per 100 ml (6–9 g/dl or 60–90 g/litre).

## HAEMOGLOBIN S/HAEMOGLOBIN C DISEASE

These people have inherited haemoglobin S from one parent and haemoglobin C from the other. They have a relatively mild form of sickle cell disease. The haemoglobin level is often normal or only slightly reduced. Levels of 11–13 g/dl are usual.

# Index